*An Inspiring Story of Love and Courage*

# SLIPPING AWAY

## One Family's Experience with a Parent's Dementia

*Luree Miller*



SIMON & SCHUSTER
AUSTRALIA

SLIPPING AWAY
First published in Australia in 1993 by
Simon & Schuster Australia
20 Barcoo Street, East Roseville NSW 2069

A Paramount Communications Company
Sydney New York London Toronto Tokyo Singapore



National Library of Australia
Cataloguing in Publication data

Miller, Luree.
Slipping away.

ISBN 0 7318 0376 0.

1. Smith, Margaret, 1892-1980 — Last years. 2. Smith family.
3. Senile dementia — Patients — United States — Biography.
4. Senile dementia — Patients — Family relationships. I. Title.

616.890092

Text design by Helen Semmler
Cover design by Kathie Baxter Smith
Typeset in Australia by Asset Typesetting Pty Ltd
Printed in Singapore by Kim Hup Lee Printing Co. Pte Limited

Born in Seattle, USA, Luree Miller has lived in Alaska, Bangladesh, India and England. A biographer, travel writer and book reviewer, she is a frequent contributor to *The Washington Post* and *The Los Angeles Times.* Her books include *Literary Hills of San Francisco, Literary Villages of London* and *Alaska: Pioneer Stories of a Twentieth Century Frontier.* She currently lives in Washington, DC.

# FOREWORD

When I read *Slipping Away*, it brought back so many memories of the illness and death of my own mother that I marvelled at the similarities of human experience. Irrespective of who we are, or where we come from, certain events in life take us past the frontiers of our own particular worlds into a universal space. Whether we mark our recognition with gravity or shout it in jubilation depends upon the event. With *Slipping Away* my response was one of deep familiarity, and gratitude that someone has had the courage and skills to write of a common human experience, but one that is frequently denied.

Most of us will have to accept the ageing of people we love. Most of us will then ourselves grow old; but when we talk crossly about "the problem" of the old, it's as though we haven't quite accepted that "the old" will one day mean us.

When you are old, any number of illnesses can bring about death, but perhaps the condition that gives us more dread than any other is loss of mind. As author Luree Miller says, "Senility is a word loaded with history and horror."

In *Slipping Away*, we experience in the most moving, intimate way the gradual loss of mind of an independent and spirited woman, Margaret Watson Smith. Marko, as she was affectionately called, suffered from multi-infarct dementia, caused by a series of small erratic strokes in her brain.

Luree Miller has written a wise and fascinating account of the illness of Marko, her mother. "Fascinating" sounds an almost ghoulish word, but I use it deliberately because the quality and clarity of writing impells, pulls you into the story, makes you weep, makes you marvel at the fierce independence of this woman whose resistance to her illness was heroic.

Parents seem all powerful. Accepting parental vulnerability is called growing up. It is never an easy process. Luree Miller takes us deep into her own reactions to her mother's illness: the fear, the irritation, the pity, the love and the guilt — the whole maelstrom of human emotions, that one by one are pulled out of Pandora's box.

No illness occurs in a vacuum — family, friend and, ultimately, society become a part of the experience. Hopefully in generations to come we will be horrified at the impersonal and therefore cruel way in which so many people are treated during institutional care — whether it is in hospital or, in this case, homes for the aged.

Miller writes, "The terrible thing is that I will never know what my mother suffered." And it is true that we can never truly know the sufferings of another. But we can be alive and open to their feelings and their fears, we can honour the dignity of their being, however ill and ravaged they become, and this is what Miller does, this and more.

These books are not easy books to write. So much that is painful and wounding, so many distressing memories, so many wonderful ones; such a cauldron of feelings comes with the kind of total honesty that this book brings us, and with such clear judgment and fine writing skill.

*Slipping Away* is not a sad book; it is a book which is a profound celebration of life, and in particular the life of Margaret Watson Smith. I thank Luree Miller for letting us share it. I wish I had read it earlier. I am glad I have read it now.

ANNE DEVESON

# CONTENTS

# 1

# NOT IN NICE FAMILIES

The death of the mind is infinitely more terrible than the death of the body and I mourned my mother that day as I was never to mourn her afterwards.

DERVLA MURPHY: *Wheels Within Wheels*

What happened happened suddenly, but that was because we had not read the signs. Looking back now, I can see that it was our pride, not just Marko's, that was the obstacle. Our insistence on her independence was a mask for our resistance to change, for her stubbornness and fear, for our ignorance. Bumbling along, we improvised, not understanding where we were going or what lay ahead. Later I learned how typical we were, how many people "suddenly" find themselves faced with husbands or wives, parents or loved ones who mysteriously have changed, who are no longer completely themselves. In subtle ways some aspects of their behaviour have altered. While we were not looking, their ability to look after themselves faltered. And then "suddenly" the world turns upside down. The unbelievable occurs. This is how it happened to us.

One cold night in mid-January Watson's phone rang. Sleepily, he answered it. A garbled voice jangled in his ear. Somebody was making gibberish sounds. Impatiently he started to hang up. Then a stab of recognition froze him. It was Marko's voice. Her tone was desperate but the words she uttered made no sense. "I'm coming!" Watson yelled into the phone. He threw on his clothes, backed his car out of the driveway between the piles of snow and sped down the dark Seattle streets to Marko's house. The shades were drawn. Several days' newspapers lay where they had been flung on the porch. The front door was locked. But he had a key and let himself in.

Hard white kernels of uncooked rice lay scattered across the living room rug. Marko appeared from the dark hallway dressed only in her summer satin nightgown. Vacantly she stared at Watson. For a moment he was too shocked to speak. She had shrunk to a skeleton. Through the thin gown he could see her bony outline. "Marko, I'm taking you to the hospital." He moved towards the hall closet, keeping an eye on her. She understood and nodded assent. Docile as a sleepy child, she let him bundle her into her heavy tweed coat and overshoes. Hurriedly he called Doctor Grant to alert the hospital, then half-carrying Marko out to his sports car, he lifted her like a rag doll into the bucket seat and fastened the safety belt across her chest.

It was nearly midnight when Watson pulled up to the emergency entrance of Mother Cabrini Hospital and dashed into Admissions. As he hurried back outside to get Marko, he saw from the bright vapour lamps of the parking lot that she was not in the car. "My God," he thought, "she's got out and she's wandering. Madison … a very busy street … even at this time of night … and all around the hospital a dark neighbourhood …" He ran to his Mercedes and there she was, slumped down so that her head was below the level of the front windshield. Walking her into the hospital was out of the question. Watson rushed back to the admissions desk to ask for a stretcher. Two orderlies brought one out of the emergency entrance and put it down on the asphalt parking lot. Effortlessly they lifted Marko's small body from the car onto the stretcher, tucked a blanket around her and bore her away between them. Watson did not see her again until the next day.

In London I answered my telephone and heard Watson say in a strained voice, "I've taken Mother to the hospital."

"Shall I come? How serious is it?" I shouted into

the bad connection. "I don't know." His voice seemed far away. "It's a case of severe malnutrition. But she's improving."

"Unbelievable!" I said to him again when I arrived in Seattle a day later. "Absolutely unbelievable. I can't understand how it happened." "I know. It doesn't seem possible." A look of anguish crossed his face. "She's just a hunk of bones. Nearly starved herself to death."

I couldn't comprehend it. My own mother nearly dying of starvation! She was not poor. She was not abandoned. But she was starving like those little old ladies you read about in the newspapers. Batty ladies, bag ladies. But not my beautiful proud mother! Utterly unbelievable! "Clothes can cover up the loss of a lot of flesh," Watson sighed. "I had absolutely no realisation of how far she had starved herself." Malnutrition, we were later told, is far more common among older people who live alone than most people realise. Even severe malnutrition like Marko was suffering from. Even when families are close by, when friends look in. Subtle physical and mental changes are seldom detected by people who see the afflicted person frequently.

In another week, on 25 January, Marko would be seventy-nine years old. She had spent Christmas with Watson, Ellen, their two daughters and five other members of Ellen's family. The celebration was noisy and Marko seemed a bit out of it. But she ate well and smiled at her granddaughters, who thought she looked quite tired. Holidays are difficult for older people, they concluded. Memories of happier times flood back. An obvious cause for Marko's silence and lack of gaiety was that she still was grieving for her husband, Virgil. Though he had been dead nearly three years, she seemed somehow still in shock, more and more withdrawn. Family and friends were getting used to her polite detachment. The period after Christmas was always a letdown and the winter was bitter. Watson, an executive at an international aircraft company, had to make several trips to Los Angeles early in January. Ellen, his wife, was stretched thin, coping with the turmoil in public education as the head of the English department in a large Seattle high school. But both kept in touch with Marko by phone. Those two weeks after Christmas Marko talked to them, to several of her friends, even to Doctor Grant. To all of them she seemed a bit depressed, as everyone was by the unusually bad weather that kept them housebound, but essentially she was her usual self. No one remembers the exact date of their last conversation with Marko before she collapsed.

So how did it happen? We will never know exactly. Much later she told me she remembered that once she woke on the kitchen floor, not sure how she got there or how long she had lain there. Her uppermost thought at the time was that she must not let Watson know because if she told him he might not let her stay on alone in her house. Perhaps that was the beginning of the small strokes that neither she nor we recognised because no obvious physical impairment lingered as a clue to the mysterious workings of her body. What was happening to her was not visually apparent. She had no classic signs of stroke: no drooping muscles in her face, no dragging gait nor weakness in her grip. Only subtle changes in her brain: the destruction of cells in her control centre, the slow death of her mind.

I didn't have the courage to go directly to the hospital to see Marko. Instead I drove to her house to leave my suitcase as I had so many times before. Her house was Home. I was the Traveller returning as I had every two years with my husband and our children on our "home leaves" from posts overseas in the United States Foreign Service. Marko's home was our base, our anchor where we enjoyed the luxuries of American life before our next posting abroad; a haven in times of troubles when one of us needed to convalesce from an illness. She prepared the children's meals when I wasn't able to and brought me coffee in bed, plumped up the pillows and pulled the curtains so I could look out on her luxuriant garden, deep green in the rain of winter or bright with summer blooms. A restful, inviting house: polished mahogany against the deep reds of her Oriental carpets, cranberry glass lamps and books on all the tables.

For several minutes I stood on the porch stamping the snow from my boots, reluctant to go in. Fumbling for the right key, I finally opened the front door. The low slanting winter sunlight streamed down the hall, lighting her brightly patterned hall carpet. As I stepped onto it, I realised the glistening dots of white were not part of the pattern; they were kernels of rice strewn the length of the runner like trail markers, leading from the living room down the hall and around the corner. Chilled and suddenly shaking, I followed the trail. It led to the door of Virgil's old study. There on his sofa was the English mohair blanket I had sent Marko last Christmas, lying like a cast-off cocoon, its blue and fuchsia plaid dotted with sprinklings of white rice. On his desk was a box of Minute Rice, what remained of its contents spilt across the large green writing blotter. Next to it was one of Marko's favourite Wedgwood cups close by the telephone. With my heart drumming in my ears, I stepped across the threshold into the study. At once the musty smell told me this is where she had lived, in Virgil's study, huddled in the mohair blanket those last days before her collapse, talking on the telephone to her family, her friends, her doctor, fooling them all so they would not take her away from her home. A spoon was stuck in the honey she had not eaten at the bottom of her cup.

I felt the pain knot in my chest move up and burst forth in wailing sobs I could not stop. Alone in my mother's house I pounded the desk and wept for her. What had she suffered here, frightened and alone? I wanted her back the way she was before.

# 2

# BEFORE WE KNEW

> Anyone can see at a glance that I am old.
> I, I alone do not see it.
>
> ELIZABETH COATSWORTH: *Personal Geography*

Nearly a decade earlier, Margaret Watson Smith, by her own choice, passed her seventieth birthday on the Gujarat Mail. Most of that nineteen-hour railway journey from Bombay to Mount Abu she spent on her knees looking out of the window because the train's wooden benches were placed parallel rather than perpendicular to the windows. Marko, as her grandchildren dubbed her and I now called her, wanted a clear view. Her camera hung round her neck and she wore no glasses. As an artist she abhorred sunglasses, even in India, because they distorted true colours. "Just look at your mother!" I remember my husband, Bill, saying, not once but a dozen times during that trip: on the train, at the crowded railway stations, as we climbed the steep hills of Mount Abu. When we explored the cool interiors of the intricately carved

Jain temples, Marko strode ahead of us in her yellow shirtwaist dress, her beautiful legs bare and unblemished. Her dark grey-brown hair was coiled in a thick braid on the crown of her head. Against the white marble pillars and pierced screens she was a tiny figure, shrunken by age to a scant five feet, but her back was so straight and her head so high that she conveyed an impression of strength and determination unrelated to size.

The whole long dusty day's journey from Mount Abu across Rajasthan to Udaipur she rode in the open jeep the way she used to sit a horse as a girl in Idaho: easily, alert, her large brown eyes watchful, her whole being infused with the blithe spirit of a traveller, who, as Marko used to say of herself, was born with sand in her shoes. This was my mother as I wanted to remember her: the eager observer, the happy traveller. "You should hope to be half as good as she is at her age," Bill had warned me — a jarring comment I quickly dismissed. In our family we generally ignored birthdays after childhood. So Marko was genuinely surprised when Bill had raised his glass to toast her at our dinner table in Bombay before we left for Mount Abu.

"Will I really be seventy tomorrow?" There was a note of wistful incredulity in her voice. "It's funny. I don't feel it."

"By God, Maggie, you're as good-looking a woman

as the day I married you," my father, Virgil, countered in a voice he hoped was gruff enough to cover the love he was embarrassed to show.

Marko reached across the table to pat his hand appreciatively. "We've seen a lot of the world together since then."

"In my judgement there's a fair amount left to investigate." Eyes twinkling, he tapped his unlit pipe and raised his eyebrows speculatively. "But I suppose you're anxious to get back to your Schoolmasters' Wives meetings and art classes."

"Now, Virgil," she cut him off. Our three children giggled at the grown-ups and fidgeted with their forks, impatient for Marko to cut her cake.

"Goodness, could you draw all of those candles?" Marko asked our youngest.

"Too many," replied eight-year-old Stacy.

Pulling a pencil from her pocket, Marko began to sketch on her paper serviette. "I'll show you how so that you don't have to draw each one separately, but line them up like this." Stacy slid out of her chair and ran around the table to poke her head up in the crook of Marko's arm. Marko handed her the pencil. The boys exchanged looks of desperation.

"You better blow the candles out, Marko. There's an awful lot of them," urged Scott.

"It's a *chocolate* cake," Blair reminded her.

"Why, I nearly forgot!" She looked up from the

drawing with an apologetic smile. "You boys help me blow out the candles." They crowded on either side of her, and, with Stacy, helped Marko pick the candles off the cake, quickly swirling each candle end in their mouths for any traces of chocolate frosting that might be clinging to its waxy surface.

I remember that scene and the flash of gratitude I felt that my children could enjoy their grandmother the way I had mine. Marko's mother had just celebrated her ninety-fifth birthday. How secure life seemed then, with my mother and my grandmother always there ahead of me.

When Marko and Virgil's visit with us in India was over, I took them to the Bombay airport, said goodbye and felt a rush of tears. I wept not for their mortality, which I did not believe in, but because again we were to be so far apart.

Five years later in Seattle, Virgil was dead. After fifty-one years of marriage Marko was a widow. Seventy-five years old. Alone. They had planned to attend a lecture on Pakistan that evening. In the morning Virgil played nine holes of golf.

That afternoon he had a cerebral haemorrhage: a massive stroke. Marko agreed to visit us in London, Bill's new post, as soon as she recovered from the shock of Virgil's death. She was staying on alone in her house. Watson and I had urged her to, confident in the knowledge that experts advised widows not to make sudden moves but to remain in familiar surroundings following their usual routines for as long as they could. Happily, Watson and Ellen lived only ten minutes away from her.

"Yes, Watson's close by," Marko agreed, putting her Wedgwood coffee cup down on the glass-topped table. She gazed out of her breakfast room window, beyond the patio and expanse of velvet green lawn to her beds of rhododendrons and azaleas: masses of magenta, salmon, pink and lavender curved around the bases of silvery firs and dark hemlocks that edged her garden. "I've worked hard on it. I don't want to give up my garden," she said determinedly.

"Be careful," I wrote to her. "Don't overtire yourself." I knew she hated to have help. She never learned to be comfortable with servants during the two years she lived in Pakistan. Being hedged in by people irritated her. She had grown up on large ranches high in the alpine meadows and pine forests of Idaho. To paint or sculpt she needed to be alone, carving out her day as inspiration moved her. Despite the distances she had travelled from the mountain ranges of the West to become first a teacher, then a faculty wife, she still was a loner, imbued with the pride and independence of a frontier woman, brave and daring, capable of adapting and improvising throughout a lifetime of enormous changes.

Watson and I applauded her individualism and her old-fashioned American virtues, confident they would serve her well in age and widowhood. We were relieved that she wanted to stay in her comfortable house with the antique furniture, the carpets and old china she had collected with discrimination and used with such pleasure. There was her garden to enjoy, her flower beds to dig in. And then, before we knew it, her insistence on independence coupled with the strength of her pride became a lethal combination. Together they almost killed her.

3

# WHEN TO BELIEVE WHAT?

> I'm going down hill — not hurrying at all, but going ... the pegs are loosening, perhaps being slowly pulled out.
>
> WALT WHITMAN from *Walt Whitman: Poet of Democracy* by Hugh L Fausset

"Cerebral arteriosclerosis" was what Doctor Grant had said when I called him before going to the hospital to see Marko. "You know your mother has suffered from it for a long time. Now, of course, her condition is complicated by malnutrition. She is hallucinating. She did not recognise a couple of old friends who came to see her. So you'd better prepare yourself for the possibility of her not recognising you. She became agitated today and threw something. Really quite confused." He paused and then went on in a low, comforting voice, "I'm sorry to say this, but Margaret will never be able to live alone again, because if she did, she would die of starvation, if nothing else. You understand, this is senile dementia. She will not get better."

"Yes, of course," was all I could say. Of course I didn't understand. I didn't even know what questions to ask.

Least of all did I know that Doctor Grant's well-meant diagnosis of cerebral arteriosclerosis was a catch-all diagnosis. Hardening of the arteries at the time he was treating Marko was considered synonymous with senile dementia. Now it is no longer tenable for a physician to diagnose a patient as senile and not make a diligent search for the causative or contributing factors. Confusion is a standard symptom of most of the ailments of the elderly. But more sophisticated clinical procedures and technical instruments make it possible to differentiate among the several dementing diseases of middle and later life. Some can be prevented, some ameliorated. All can be treated with more understanding.

Senility is a word loaded with history and horror. It should not be used without a careful explanation. Shakespeare's seven stages of man haunt us and shape our expectations. The last stage is "second childishness and mere oblivion". But that was in the sixteenth century, when nutrition and sanitation and all of the sciences that contribute to our well-being were in their infancy. Medical and psychological studies have proved that old age need not be a time of diminishing mental capacities. Yet the whisper of it in one's own family creates such a profound anxiety it is next to impossible to think clearly. Few things are more terrifying than the fear of mental incompetence. If it were happening to my mother, my subconscious said, it would happen to me. I squelched the thought, but not the anxiety. It kept me off balance when I should have been most lucid and rational.

"It is sad but inevitable," Doctor Grant had told me the year before when I asked his advice about Marko's problems with the various help we had arranged for her. "All old people decline mentally and some become difficult," he declared. Then he had leaned across the wide desk between us. "But your father," he said, "was more disciplined than your mother, so his slippage was not so apparent." I remember my chagrin and the shared guilt I felt with Marko for being an "undisciplined" woman, she an artist, I a writer. Doctor Grant shrugged his shoulders and smiled. His message was clear With the application of a little will-power and self-discipline as my father had, she could manage her life better, though of course the trend was irrevocably downward.

Now I wonder if he were one of the doctors who call older women "female crocks" and dismiss their complaints as attention-getting strategies not worthy of a busy doctor's consideration. Did he take the time to observe that the loss of Virgil, her husband of more than fifty years, might have been too profound for her to overcome at her age? Did he suspect that an underlying depression might be contributing to her intellectual deterioration? Now more doctors know that depression is increasingly identified as one of the bases for impaired mental function in older people. They recognise that depressed people often deny their despondent feelings, particularly those of Marko's generation who were brought up believing emotional states to be entirely within their control. So rather than talk about feelings, they focus on bodily complaints.

Doctor Grant must have accepted her litany of physical complaints at face value. He must not have considered that she might have an undercurrent of mental anguish. Or questioned her ability to take medications as he directed. She had bottles and bottles of prescription pills. It is difficult, now that the public's attention has been drawn to the dangers of excessive and inappropriate drug prescriptions for older people, not to feel that Marko suffered also from excessive drug use. It was a joke in our family that a half glass of wine made her tipsy. She was sensitive to foods and drugs, and like most people, probably became more so as she grew older.

When I looked in her medicine cabinet that cold winter day before I went to see her in the hospital, I found it filled with prescription drugs. If Doctor Grant thought she were slipping mentally, why did he prescribe so many pills? How could she have remembered which ones she took and when? How many had she swallowed in desperation, confusedly reaching for something to lift the cloud, to make her feel well again? Now it is known that the elderly who suffer from arteriosclerosis usually show a negative response to even small amounts of drugs. Those who are undernourished as well may have exaggerated drug reactions. Marko's anti-hypertension medication may have created more symptoms than it alleviated.

Like many older people, Marko's total physical status was complicated: depression, too many drugs, first not eating the right foods (the common "tea and toast syndrome"), then not eating at all. Add to that her history of hypertension or high blood pressure. But like most family members of an afflicted person, I was both too ignorant of medicine and psychology and too emotionally upset to sort out the symptoms or understand the implications of her condition.

I waited alone that day in Marko's house until evening visiting hours before I had the courage to go to the hospital to see her. A nurse at the desk on the fifth floor gave me her room number and as an afterthought added, "She's been restrained, but I don't think she is now."

"She's been what?" I asked.

"Restrained." The nurse eyed me steadily. "She kept getting up and wandering. Earlier today she threw a box of candy at a nurse. We had to tie her hands to the side of the bed. I think she's untied now."

Too appalled to answer, I hurried down the wide hospital corridor to Marko's room, my heart pounding. Her bed was empty. But she was standing beside it in a white hospital gown on the opposite side facing the door. Her face was gaunt. Frowning, she smoothed the sheets, running her hands up under the pillow. In that instant when she first glanced up I saw in her great brown eyes a haunted look like that of a frightened animal. Then she focused on me. At once her face lit up with a smile of delight. "Darling!" she gasped. I rushed around the end of the bed to throw my arms around her. "Marko, Marko," I cried. We clung to each other, rocking back and forth, until finally I pulled away and helped her back into bed.

"What have you done, Marko?" I asked her. "They say you threw something."

She pursed her lips and narrowed her eyes, looking at me closely. Then she leaned forward and whispered, "Hope came to see me."

"Really?" I was surprised. Hope was a sister-in-law she had resented for fifty years. They avoided each other assiduously.

"Oh yes. She came!" Marko grabbed my arm. An expression of glee flicked across her face. "Hope came and just stood there at the foot of my bed. So I picked up a box of candy and aimed for her head."

"Did you hit her?"

"Yes, of course. Right in the face. Did she yell!" Marko gave a sigh of satisfaction and lay back on the pillow smiling happily. "I've always had a good eye."

I saw that she was waiting for me to congratulate her. "Well, good for you," I said. "Good aim." And I burst out laughing.

"Got her at last," Marko grinned. She began to laugh too. Neither of us could stop. It was as if we were poised together at the top of a roller-coaster, clinging to each other, scared and giggling helplessly before our next swoop downward.

# 4

# FAULTY CONNECTIONS

> I made feeble attempts at signalling the plight into which I had come, but in the noise and turmoil of the world, these were not noticed.
>
> GUY WINT: *The Third Killer*

The terrible thing is that I will never know what Marko suffered. I will never know what she felt or what she thought. Too many complications had weakened her body and clouded her mind. She was not like someone with fractured ribs who can point to an area of pain and tell how it feels. She could not describe what had happened to her. And nothing in my experience enabled me to imagine her state of mind. It was too late for rational communication between us.

Yet she was alive. She would go on living. What I desperately needed to know was what had happened to her and what could be done. That understanding was painfully slow in coming. Had I understood what was happening, it could have relieved some of the tension and spared all of us the crushing weight of misplaced blame and guilt. For now, in retrospect, it seems clear that Marko first suffered from a series of "little strokes" later complicated by severe depression, possible drug intoxication, and the malnutrition that finally caused her to collapse. What happened to her is all too typical in older people who, however loved, are still without advocates to insist their doctors pay attention and their families understand.

There were early warning signs: her complaints of dizziness or sudden confusion or headaches; her vague physical complaints; the time she felt a wave of "sickness" so severe she dropped her trowel and staggered to a *chaise longue,* flopping stretched out until the sick feeling passed. All of these symptoms had gone on for years. We didn't understand their cause and their steady recurrence dulled our concern. Because Marko was basically sturdy, she snapped back from any of these temporary indispositions to work long hours sculpting or gardening. By her resumption of vigorous activity she dispelled any suspicions we might have had that her complaints were important clues leading to a later devastating illness. Had we seen it coming, we could have watched her more closely, been more prepared. We would have known that each little stroke destroys a small area of brain tissue, that a continuation of these mini-strokes causes an irreversible dementia called multi-infarct dementia. (*Infarct* is the medical term for a stroke.)

Instead we were irritated with Marko when she fought with the cleaning woman and did not pay her bills on time; when she insisted that the neighbours were turning off her outdoor lights.

It was not her fault. Her brain was being destroyed bit by bit. She was being treated for hypertension, or high blood pressure, which often causes these "little strokes". But the treatment of hypertension in older people is itself hazardous because over-treatment can also contribute to brain damage.

"Little strokes" are medically termed *transient ischemic attacks* or TIAs. Transient refers to the fact that they last a very short time, anywhere from two to thirty minutes and never beyond twenty-four hours. They are transient rather than completed strokes. The symptoms pass. The victim returns to normal, or seems to. No paralysis or loss of speech results as in a completed stroke. The damage is hidden in the enormous complexity of the brain.

Ischemic means a localised tissue anaemia. An obstruction in the arterial blood flow may occur: a blocking of a blood vessel by a small blood clot or a bubble of air. Or a small blood vessel may burst, haemorrhaging into the brain. This temporary interference with the blood supply to a specific area of the brain causes the vertigo or wave of nausea, a slurring of the speech, or a numbness in a limb typical of TIAs. Or the stroke may be so small as to go entirely unnoticed. A major stroke is quite different. Then a large blood vessel is involved and the symptoms are sudden, dramatic, and sometimes fatal.

TIAs usually are the harbingers of major disabling or fatal cerebral infarctions or strokes. Relentlessly they attacked Marko until finally a massive stroke caused her death. In the decade between her collapse and her death we ran the gamut of anguishing problems that devastate families coping with an older member's increasing dementia.

Dementia or deteriorating mental ability does not occur swiftly and dramatically like a heart attack. It does not galvanise the family into action. It creeps like crab grass until one day the balance between healthy lawn and straggly weed is so apparent you can no longer ignore it.

Slowly and silently these "little strokes" altered Marko's personality and interfered with her ability to think rationally or to carry out simple motor functions. Yet, for a long time, Marko's strong will and tremendous capacity to compensate deceived us.

Christmas Day when Watson picked her up for dinner she was immaculately dressed in her best brocade suit, her black suede gloves matching her shoes and bag, her long hair carefully done up. Who would have guessed that in her bedroom were the Christmas packages she had received from her sisters, her friends, and me, all unopened? I found them later lying on the floor beside her unmade bed. She had clawed at the strings and wrapping paper but somehow had not been able to tear the wrappings off. On her rumpled sheets were Christmas cards she had written on, over and over, the same phrase, "Dearest Luree". The message was never completed; the cards never sent.

Victims of major strokes who are fortunate to have recovered sufficiently to remember and record their experiences testify that they had the illusion they were perfectly clear in their minds when by their actions it was apparent they were not. Marko must have felt this way, at least in the beginning. And so in those days before her hospitalisation we argued with her as we argued with each other. We told her that she must have more help, or get someone to live with her, or move out of her house to an apartment that would be easier for her to care for. Our arguments were rational and logical. Fiercely she rejected them all. "She's hopelessly stubborn," we said. "She won't listen to reason."

But how can the mind know that it is not working properly? How can it be aware that microscopic abnormalities are affecting its intellectual functioning? That TIAs are short-circuiting its synapses?

Multi-infarct dementia caused by TIAs is one of the more than fifty causes of irreversible dementia among older people. Most common is Alzheimer's disease, a cerebral degenerative disorder of unknown cause which also causes dementia. The end stages of both diseases, Alzheimer's and multi-infarct dementia, are the same. Both result in severe dementia and death. But the clinical processes or progression of the two diseases are crucially different. Alzheimer's victims deteriorate in an overall, steadily progressive pattern. They are the patients we think of as classically senile.

Those who suffer from multi-infarct dementia have a spotty, step-like, erratic deterioration. Like a random pin-pricking of a cluster of balloons, the little strokes destroy tiny areas of brain tissue. In each person the affected areas are different, so the behavioural changes are unpredictable. The special agony of TIA victims is that eventually, when their bodies will not obey their mental orders, they know something terrible and frightening, something beyond their control, is happening. This stage of their dementia, when they can comprehend they are losing control, is terrifying. Nobody notices. Nobody understands. Because the specialists at the hospital, after running Marko through extensive and expensive tests, told us without qualifications or specifics, that she was becoming senile, we fell into the habit of not really paying attention to her. We treated her more and more as if she were simply not there. Following the lead of doctors and nurses, our tone became slightly patronising. Then one day several years after her collapse, Marko came into my kitchen to ask if she could help with dinner. I counted out the silverware and gave it to her to set the table. She went into the dining room. After a while I noticed that she had been gone a long time and that I had not heard her moving about. I went to investigate.

Marko was standing rigidly at the head of the table. Her arms were bent upwards like a wooden soldier's. In one hand she clutched the knives and forks, in the other the spoons. "Marko, what's the matter?" I cried.

She did not move. A look of terror lit her eyes. I started toward her. She shook her head. I waited. Some fierce internal struggle held her motionless. Then her arms dropped to the table, her hands still clutching the silverware.

"My mind," she said very slowly and clearly, "can't make my hands do what my eyes see."

Her face was filled with fright. She was a prisoner in her own body. She was no longer in control and she knew it. Her damaged brain could not activate that wave of electrochemical activity needed to transmit a nerve impulse to the needed muscle. It was the problem of the stroke victim. If her body would not always obey her, then her speech must not always reflect her thoughts. How often had she tried to say what she was thinking and been unable to command her words? What a struggle, what strength of will it cost her to produce that brilliant summary of her condition: "My mind can't make my hands do what my eyes see."

Marko's *cri de coeur* jolted me into awareness. She was not "senile" in the simplistic sense that I had always understood it: a doddery old person with a benign loss of mental faculties. Anguish and frustration racked her. Bit by bit her control was being cut off. Every TIA diminished her.

But *she* was there. Thinking, feeling, suffering. I vowed from that time forward never to forget, however severed our lines of communication might become, that the essence of Marko was alive within her, trapped, yet aware. But that insight and my resolve came after years of impatience, anger, guilt and despair.

5

# THE DREADED DECISION IS MADE

> Ask me no more: thy fate and mine are seal'd:
> I strove against the stream and all in vain
>
> ALFRED, LORD TENNYSON: *The Princess*

"Under no circumstances should you look at nursing homes by yourself," Irene said. "I'm taking you. Remember, I've been through it all myself and I know what it's like. It's not easy. You have to prepare yourself. The way it works is we go in and look at a home. Then we come back out to the car and cry a bit. Then we look at another one and come out and cry. That's just the way it goes. But first, let's have lunch."

Practical, honest, down-to-earth Irene was a friend I was blessed to have at this time in this place. Marko had been in the hospital three weeks. Doctor Grant said she would have to be transferred to a nursing home, that there was no question of her returning to her own home. She would need twenty-four-hour care because of her disorientation and her sudden wanderings. Her paranoia had increased. As strength flowed back into her frail body she flayed at the nurses and scorned the doctors. In the hospital setting Watson and I were able to view Marko with an objectivity we could never have achieved while she was at home. There she was mistress of her own house and our mother. She ignored our advice and did as she wished. While she was in the hospital we had a breather to digest the dismal prognosis Doctor Grant gave us: patients with cerebral arteriosclerosis generally move from paranoia to combativeness to agitation to compulsive behaviour, exhibiting all tendencies in varying degrees of severity.

Even though I now know that cerebral arteriosclerosis is a general, imprecise diagnosis, it is true that most patients suffering mental deterioration develop these symptoms, especially paranoia. Perhaps anxiety and fear are the basis of their paranoia — a terrifying sense of not being able to look after themselves as they once could, of being vulnerable. Marko, always a night owl, had begun staying up all night. Alone in her house for the first time in her entire life, it must have been too frightening for her to switch off the lights and lie down in the dark listening to the night sounds. Safer to sleep by day.

I deplored this warped behaviour but never thought

of it as evidence of a basic personality change taking place in Marko. Shame and humiliation at having my mother show signs of mental deterioration must have made me cover up for her irrationality. We became used to her odd behaviour, to her complaints. We never realised that many of the tendencies she was developing were symptoms typical of multi-infarct dementia: her irritability and confusion and her clinging to absurd delusions.

One moment I was certain that she really was having delusions, the next an explanation emerged for some bizarre coincidence. It kept Watson and me continually off-balance. She was convinced that the paper boy was putting pins in the doorbell which set off a terrible ringing in her ears. When next she complained that her garage door opened mysteriously every morning and night so that she had to run out and close it, we were certain she was making it all up. Then the neighbour across the street called to apologise: the remote control device in his car was operating on the same frequency as Marko's, opening not only his garage door, but hers too. How then could we say the paper boy was not putting pins in her doorbell, since she failed to tip him as Virgil always had? When she accused the cleaning women we hired for her of stealing her jewellery, breaking her china, or scrubbing her oil painting with a wire brush, there was no way for us to sort fact from fiction before she fired them.

"You're lucky," Irene said. "The doctor has made the decision for you. Most people don't have such a clear-cut situation when they finally have to put someone in a nursing home. They muddle along, hoping they can manage somehow. They try everything to keep the person at home until one day something left on the stove catches fire or the person wanders off and gets lost like mother did. It was six hours before we found her wandering along a country road."

I had visions of Marko, confused and panicking, in the crush of traffic on Oxford Street where we lived. Still I wavered. "Maybe I should take her to London to live with me. I know that's what she would like best." In the hospital Marko had whispered, "Why can't I live with you? Louise took care of Mother." The dreaded question. I flushed with guilt. "Aunt Louise had no children and she lived in a little town in Idaho," I replied, knowing it was an answer for me, not for her — knowing that more than anything else she wanted to be with me and Bill and our children. Instinctively she grasped for life, against the isolation of the institution I would be delivering her to. I felt as if I were pushing her out of my lifeboat.

"I know how you feel, but you've got to be reasonable." Irene pulled her car keys out of her bag and stood up. "You couldn't look after her properly. She could never be left alone. She would drive you all crazy and you wouldn't really be doing her any good. Remember, you've a husband and children to take care of. Think of them. Come on. Let's go."

Grateful for her certainty, I followed. But both love and guilt compelled me to keep considering how I might take Marko with me.

"You have to develop a perspective," Irene argued. "I remember one day when I was getting a big family dinner. My mother was pretty confused by this time and believe me, so was I. What I took out of the refrigerator, she put back in. Same with dirty dishes. She stuffed them in the cupboard as fast as she found them and got furious if I tried to stop her. Then she went outside and started pulling up all of the plants as if they were weeds. The last straw was when Mother looked straight at me and said, 'Well, I certainly enjoyed having all of you over, but I do worry about Irene. I wonder what's happened to her.' "

I laughed and Irene shrugged her shoulders. "It's a terrible thing to go through." Her voice was full of sympathy. "I know. But your mother will probably let go of you sooner and more easily than you will let go of her." As we walked up the path to another nursing home, I took Irene's arm, acutely aware that one of the greatest gifts anyone can have in a time of crisis is a sensible friend who can show you the road ahead.

Selecting a nursing home under duress is the worst possible way to view one. I hated the whole idea of nursing homes because they represented failure — failure on my part to solve the problems of my mother's loneliness and her progressive dementia. This feeling of failure was reinforced by Marko's friends, who expressed surprise and disapproval that I would even consider a nursing home for her. "I'm sure she'll be just fine in no time," they said. "She loves her home so much. She'll recover more quickly there than anywhere." Unable yet to fully accept the inevitability of her condition, I couldn't bring myself to bluntly tell her contemporaries that she would never be well enough to look after herself again, and the hints that I dropped to that effect they never picked up. In their eyes I was the villain, the ungrateful daughter.

I shifted my anger at Marko's plight onto the nursing homes. Because I hated to see her deteriorate and could do nothing about it, I hated the nursing homes that represented her decline. Without Irene to constantly point out the fact that professionally trained people could care for Marko with medical understanding and facilities I could not provide, I doubt if I could have faced the selection process.

It is a shock to see the nursing care sections: rooms full of old people with canes or walkers or in wheelchairs. Some are staring vacantly, others drooling, some moaning. It is like being dropped suddenly into another country where not just a few, but all of the inhabitants are wrinkled with age, bent and shuffling, or bedridden with some terrible affliction. Mortality en masse. No wonder I cried in the car after each visit. I cried for the fate of all those ill old people and for the fact that my own mother was now one of them.

The nursing home I finally chose was bright and sunny. There was a garden Marko could work in if she wanted to, plenty of activities for the residents, and she could bring her own furniture except for the bed and rugs. It seemed superior in all respects, with a consideration for the individuality of the patients that other nursing homes lacked. One of the main reasons I chose the North End Nursing Home was because it did not require Marko to cut her waist-length hair. The others did. "For convenience and cleanliness." The admissions directors all smiled. "You understand, I'm sure." What I understood was that they rated staff convenience higher than the patient's personal preference and pride, and that a good deal of regimentation would be rationalised as necessary for cleanliness.

Marko had "bobbed" her hair in the twenties and I grew up on the story of how Virgil first flew into a rage when he saw her shorn of the thick brown braid she wound round her head. Then he begged her to let her hair grow long again. Not until Watson and

I were gone from home did she decide to please him in this respect. Belated as it was, Virgil was happy and Marko proud that in her sixties and seventies her hair was still silky and heavy. Sitting on a low stool on our verandah in Bombay, she had let Stacy brush and drape it like a *burkha* over her face and shoulders. To cut her hair now that so much was being taken away from her would have been cruel in the extreme. At North End they understood this.

Typical of Seattle, it was raining the day an ambulance brought Marko to the nursing home. Two burly young orderlies lifted her off the stretcher onto her rolled-up hospital bed and I tucked her in. "Well, this *is* an improvement," she said. She smiled and I watched her quickly take inventory of the room. In front of a large picture window where she could see the tops of fir trees, I had placed the two wing-back chairs from her living room, her Pembroke table between them. Opposite the end of her bed was her bow-front bureau with the big bevel-edged mirror above it. I had hung as many of her pictures as the walls would take.

"You're here to convalesce," I told Marko as Doctor Grant had suggested. For a while I think she believed her stay was temporary. My deceit troubled me but there was no way in the world I would have had the courage to tell her flat out that she was here to stay. Such finality was too raw a truth for either of us to handle.

The first night she bit the nurse who thought she wore dentures and insisted that she take them out. Or so Marko told me, thereby emphasising how different she was from the others at the North End. She still had all of her own teeth — and she could bite.

In the beginning Marko revelled in the attention she received. An aide, a Norwegian woman named Tilla, greatly admired her hair. Tilla brushed it carefully, braided it beautifully and could do it up in several attractive styles. My hopes were high that Marko would settle in and soon be strong enough to participate in the home's activities.

North End was only five blocks from Marko's house. For over a month I shuttled that short distance between her two such different worlds. My daily agony was dismantling Marko's house. I was packing up her life, not knowing what to do with vestiges of an era now ended: stacks of hand-embroidered place-mats and heavy linen tablecloths she used to dampen and roll in bath towels, then iron on the dining room table; crystal goblets too fragile for the dishwasher; dresses, hats and shoes long out of fashion. Once in a burst of anguish I pushed aside Marko's dried-up paints and stiff brushes and grabbed her sketching pad to scribble myself a stern warning: 'Get yourself to a retirement home before your mind is gone, while you can still make a choice.' I was thinking of the Hindus who recognise the stages of life humans pass through and prescribe conduct for each of them. In the last stage, divestment of worldly possessions is thought proper in order to have freedom and time to contemplate the mysteries of life and seek oneness with the universe. How opposite from the American way. We want to stay young and independent, surrounded by more possessions than we can possibly use or care for, doing the same things we've always done. Prisoners of our possessions; slaves to them. Defying nature. Making age a tragedy and failure.

As I packed box after box of woollens Marko hadn't worn in years, lengths of cloth she had never made up, and Virgil's clothes that had hung for three years in the closet, Emily Dickinson's poem kept running through my head:

The Bustle in a House
The Morning after Death
Is solemnest of industries
Enacted upon Earth —

The sweeping up the Heart
And putting Love away
We shall not want to use again
Until Eternity.

Only Marko was not dead. "Look in my chiffonier, in the bottom drawer under my scarves and you'll find a book of traveller's cheques," she instructed me. I couldn't find them. Watson and Ellen helped me on weekends and once Scott came up from Reed College in Portland. "What's this?" he asked as he picked an ivory-handled button hook out of a box of sculpting tools. In a trunk still fragrant with lavender I found unfinished needlepoint canvases rolled in yellowed newspapers dated the year I was born. Silently we stacked and sorted and packed. "I'll miss this house," Scott sighed. We looked out of the front windows, across Puget Sound to Agate Pass and the snow-capped Olympic Mountains beyond. Scott patted my shoulder.

After the house was empty, the electricity turned off, and I was locking up for the last time, Marko's sister, Louise, suddenly remembered. "Did you pull out the kitchen drawers? Mother used to hide things behind them. Maybe Margaret did too."

We raced back into the darkening kitchen, hurriedly pulling out one cabinet drawer after another. Behind the third one down my fingers touched something and I pulled out a long thin jewellery box. In the failing light I read, on the top of the box in Marko's beautiful flowing script, "For Luree and Stacy." Shakily I opened the lid. There, in the folds of tissue paper, were a delicate pin set with an amethyst and pearls, a wide gold wedding band and the signet ring my grandmother always wore with her initials, L.T., intertwined in a Victorian design. Stuffed through the gold band was a scrap of paper. Unfolding it I was startled to see the date Marko had written at the top:

"Oct. 1962." Nearly ten years ago! Or could she have got the date wrong? Her note read: "While I'm still in my right mind I want to give you, Luree, my mother's favourite pin, her wedding ring and the signet ring Papa gave her. Wear them and enjoy them as much as I have. When I'm gone they're yours and you pass them on to Stacy."

So Marko did know! She had felt herself slipping. She had begun her divestment. Labelling her small treasures, selecting pieces imbued with family history, and making her notes, she had begun the process of relinquishing and passing on. But too late. Standing in her now darkened kitchen I felt a rush of terror that made my spine tingle, my palms damp — the kind of terror she must have fought against — the chilling sense of slipping away that made her hide her treasures and write her warning: "While I'm still in my right mind …"

"I found some of Grammie's jewellery," I told Marko the next day. Her face brightened. "Oh, where?" she asked.

In the nursing home Marko was beginning to lose her tense expression, to laugh with her old abandon. "I like this second floor room," she said, looking out of the window. "I feel safe like I did in our upstairs bedroom in the old house."

"She'll never be able to move downstairs to the retirement level," the North End nurses told me. "She's lost all sense of time, forgets where she is and sometimes gets quite agitated."

Still, I went back to London hopeful that she would be happier, knowing she would be fed and properly cared for. Ellen, even though she worked full-time and had two older parents of her own, assumed the responsibility, as women traditionally do. She visited Marko regularly and arranged for someone to take her to the doctor and on outings. She looked after Marko's clothes and toiletries, brought her plants and flowers, and urged her to talk about her childhood in Idaho. And she wrote me reports. Ellen and I had always been close, now more than ever, and I was grateful beyond words to her. Watson visited less often, to have her sign cheques and to adjust her television. He didn't know what to say to her.

One spring day after the long cold winter, when the sun was pouring in through the big windows of the North End Nursing Home, Marko walked off exactly as Irene's mother had. There is no way of knowing if she wandered about her old neighbourhood finding her way by chance or if she went straight to her house. In either case she must have walked up the front path, looked in the curtainless windows and seen the bare rooms. The house was empty and locked. But no lock barred the gate to the back garden. Marko pushed the gate open and found a broken trowel. On her hands and knees she dug slowly round her flower beds until dusk when a nursing home aide found her.

"She's not happy," Ellen wrote. "There seems to be nothing that we can do about it."

"Is she strong enough to travel?" I queried Doctor Grant. He replied, "I'll let you know when she can. I think it would do her good."

That autumn Blair entered the University of Washington in Seattle. Marko began saving tea bags, sugar, salt and pepper packs, rubber bands, toothpicks, paper napkins, newspapers and magazines for him. She stuffed her purses, her drawers, and her closets. The fire inspector complained. Tilla tried to clean out the newspapers. Marko hit her. "Mrs Smith can be so sweet. But sometimes she has an awful temper." Tilla shook her head.

"She has no privacy," Blair declared. "That's the worst thing. Anybody can walk into her room anytime. They tell her when to eat, when to take a bath, when to go to bed. No wonder she's getting fed up and is fighting with everyone. I would be too."

"Ask her if she wants to come to London with you for Christmas," I wrote to him.

"She's packing her bags already," Blair called back. "I told her we would fly over the North Pole and she's so excited the nurses say she's been up and dressed and ready to go every morning since I told her. She hasn't forgotten a word I said. She repeats it to them all the time. At this rate she'll be worn out before we leave.'

A month later Marko and Blair arrived at Heathrow Airport, as incongruous a pair as ever passed through British customs: Marko, a well-dressed little figure in her new red coat and smart black hat, proud, erect, every inch a lady, on the arm of Blair, with beard and backpack, in leather jacket and shaggy fur hat. Both were beaming. "It was fun, wasn't it, Marko?" He hugged her gently.

"Absolutely wonderful. A beautiful moonlight flight." She squeezed his hand and smiled up at him. Then, to me, she flashed a look of triumph, a stubborn, defiant smile that suddenly made my stomach knot. She had escaped. Marko was travelling once again.

# 6

# A TRAVELLER STILL

Without memory there is no person.

AGNES DE MILLE: *Reprieve*

Not knowing what to expect, we were a little afraid of Marko. Tensions are contagious and Marko was tense, fierce, and restless. Roaming from room to room she would startle Bill or me and whoever might happen to be with us by throwing out the challenge, "Who says these are my golden years?" None of us ever knew how to answer her.

At this time entertaining was an aspect of Bill's work that I shared. Marko had filled the same role being hostess for Virgil's colleagues and she seemed pleased when I told her we were going to give a party. The next thing I knew she had climbed on to the dining room table to wash the crystal chandelier. "Leave me alone," she commanded when I rushed to get her down. "I'm not going to fall. This chandelier is filthy and *I* want it to shine." She glared at me. "You won't take the trouble because you're always writing."

What can a slothful daughter say to a righteous mother? My Swiss grandmother had raised Marko on the dictum, "Cleanliness is next to godliness." Marko passed the teaching along to me. No frivolous reading of books until the house shines and all the clothes are clean. It was an old argument full of resentment on my part and rage on hers.

Troubling me even more was the thought of what she would say to my British guests, most of whom I was meeting for the first time. In a small family setting it was difficult enough to cope with Marko's outbursts. She had flared at Stacy for casually mentioning at the dinner table that the Spaniards introduced horses to the New World. "Oh no they didn't," Marko snapped. "The Indians did. Chief Joseph told me so." Stacy made a mild protest. Marko became angry and excited. Our dinner was cold before we quieted her down.

What if she were incited by a guest's remark? Should I warn them? What could I do? "You have to learn to laugh," I remember Irene counselling me. "It's all that saves your sanity."

I thought of greeting each guest at the door with a whispered aside: "My mother is slightly dotty so please don't mind her. And try not to set her off, would you? She's particularly sensitive on the subjects of Red Indians, horses, abstract painting, modern sculpture, antique furniture, Oriental rugs, old china, synthetics, schoolteachers, politics, taxes, child rearing, old age, travel and gardening.'

Wistfully I remembered a party in India where the hostess took each guest over to meet her mother sitting on a charpoy like an Oriental queen receiving courtiers, honoured, included, but without conversational demands made upon her.

The night of the party Marko seemed in a serene mood. As I passed the canapés she conversed animatedly with a man from the BBC and his stunning young wife. Marko's eyes shone, her manner was that of an experienced hostess. The BBC man moved on while his wife continued talking with Marko. I stopped to ask if she would like something to drink. Impatiently Marko waved me away. "Don't bother us now," she said. "We're having a wonderful conversation about gardening. Mrs K — has a rock garden too and we grow many of the same plants." Marko turned back to Mrs K — with a gracious smile. "Since our climate in Seattle is much the same as yours in London, I'm sure that primulas would do well for you too," she said. "After all, the vulgaris is the true English primrose, isn't it? Why don't you try some for a touch of colour? Their yellow next to a grey granite rock is a lovely contrast. I like to keep my rock garden neat and vacuumed," she continued with enthusiasm. "The vacuum picks up rocks though — with an awful racket. I can hear them rattle around in my head. Sometimes the noise goes on all day. It drives me wild. And a vacuum is hard to handle in a rock garden, don't you think?"

"Oh, quite," I heard Mrs K — respond in a rather desperate tone before I fled to the far side of the room.

When I had recovered enough to gather up my courage, I started back to deflect Marko from the beleaguered Mrs K —. Marko saw me coming and her eyes took on the wary expression of a puppy or small child who knows they are doing something wrong and will be removed. Would she bite or run? Cautiously I moved towards her and slowly she began to back away. I manoeuvred her across the hall, into the kitchen, closed the door, and started to say, "Marko, you mustn't ..." But there she stood, helpless before me, her face and body drooping with bewilderment.

"I think I'm losing my marbles," she said. Tears welled in her eyes.

I folded her into my arms. "Don't worry, Marko. It's all right," I lied, for what was there to say?

Marko's depression deepened, unrelenting, all-pervasive, until those traces of her quick wit and sharp observations were buried and lost beneath the black fog. She began to wear an expression of constant woe, her passivity interrupted only by episodes of extreme agitation or anger. Her presence cast a pall over everyone. The sharp contrast between her life and ours made me feel guilty. Here we were full of enthusiasm at being in London, one of our most stimulating posts in the Foreign Service, a marvellous city for Stacy, Blair and Scott, now in their teens. They rushed in and out glowing with excitement and discovery. Bill relished his work. Editors offered me assignments. The phone rang for all of us. Marko slumped in her chair. "I'm losing my marbles," she said over and over.

Without protest she flew back to Seattle with Blair and returned to the North End Nursing Home. Watson and I had to face the fact that her mental decline was slow and her body sturdy so that she probably would live a long time. If she had inherited her mother's genes she was programmed into her late nineties. At eighty that gave her well over a decade to go. With the increasing rate of inflation and rising nursing home costs, there was no way her money would last as long as she did. We knew that if we had to take on the full cost of her care it would be a severe financial burden. But rather than cut back on her care to make her money last longer, we decided to choose the best we could find and gamble on the future. But from this point forward, the worry about her finances settled down on us, a constant, nagging concern, another factor to consider in all of the other family decisions we made. Buying private care was a high-stakes gamble on a short future for Marko.

The North End Nursing Home was expensive; it seemed the best. But it turned out that for Marko it was not.

Unlike senile dementia of the classic Alzheimer's type, Marko's multi-infarct dementia did not render her oblivious to her surroundings. She was confused. Her sense of time, never strong even before her TIAs, was completely gone. And she had memory losses and odd aberrations in her reasoning processes. Occasionally delusions, such as insisting that she had to meet her long-dead brother, Tom, made her wildly excited. But she was never confused about who the people around her were or where she was living.

Haughtily she resisted all efforts by the nurses and aides at North End to include her in the home's activities. How could she, an artist who had studied with Mark Tobey and exhibited in the Henry Art Gallery, go to the arts and crafts groups where they painted brick door stops and made rag dolls? Those people shuffling down the halls in their slippers or sitting lined up in wheelchairs she would not accept as her colleagues.

The nurses deplored her resistance and pushed her to join in. Now I know that by then the TIAs had destroyed much of Marko's mental control over her fine motor coordination. Once a skilled knitter who would knit suits for herself, she no longer was able to send her hands messages on how to control the needles. She could not paint or draw. Mind-to-hand communication for these skills was severed. Her visual-motor functioning was impaired. The more we pushed her, the more anxious and irritable she became — a classic, predictable reaction we didn't understand. This standard problem is called a Goldstein catastrophic reaction and described as "the tendency of the brain-damaged to flood with anxiety when confronted with a task they cannot handle". In our ignorance (and that of the nursing home staff) we were trying to stimulate her beyond her capacity. It only aggravated her and irritated us. She could button her blouse, butter her bread, cut her meat and write her name. So why, we all reasoned, wouldn't she paint or sculpt?

The special agony of the TIA victim is that she can't tell you why. And the pattern of her deterioration is so erratic, so spotty and illogical, that her behaviour is a skein of contradictions.

The only constant at this time was her paranoia. Everyone in the home, she complained, was stealing from her. Of all the problems besetting chronically brain-damaged people, the most distressing to deal with is paranoia. Logic, reassurance, even the recovery of the supposedly lost item is no consolation to the paranoid person. Doctor Grant prescribed an antidepressant and wrote to me that he would "manipulate her medication" to the best effect.

Marko's paranoia coupled with her depression

hardly made her a happy person to visit. Her oldest, dearest friend confessed that Marko's endless accusations and complaints were more than she could bear, so she scarcely saw Marko any more. Other old friends faded away. Many, like herself, were in retirement or nursing homes. Many had died. Keeping her in Seattle because of her friends and the fact that it had been her home for fifty years no longer meant that much.

Management and personnel at North End changed too. A smell of urine began to pervade the halls. Marko had entered North End as Mrs Smith, a woman of some dignity who was treated with respect and consideration. Slowly she became Marko to nurses she didn't know and to aides young enough to be her grandchildren. Such intimacy was an affront to a woman of her generation. They patted her arm and treated her like a child. I felt her seethe but she couldn't muster the words that would have put them in their places. Then, on one of my periodic visits to Seattle, a head nurse told me how they "handled" her. One night when Marko refused to go to dinner, the nurse informed her that if she didn't come they would get a wheelchair and wheel her into the dining room. The threat worked. Marko went to dinner. I could imagine her walking down the hall, head high, mouth set, hating them all.

A wheelchair was a symbol of defeat for Marko. When she and Blair flew to London for holidays or summer visits, we urged her to let us send a wheelchair to the plane so she wouldn't have to walk through the long corridors of Heathrow Airport. But she always refused. After the nine-hour, all-night flight, she walked their dreary length holding Blair's arm. Patiently he kept pace with her, proud of his grandmother's pride.

We understood her fierce independence, her quirks, her references. But her increasing inability to give a clear account of her feelings and physical problems was putting her more and more at the mercy of nurses and aides who couldn't guess, as I could, what she might need or want. Her references were becoming more allusive, reasonable only to those of us close to her.

A person with waning intelligence needs the security of knowing someone is paying attention and understands.

"My slides!" Marko said, grabbing my arm.

"I took them out of the hall chest," I assured her, "and put the ones you took in Pakistan in separate boxes."

She sighed with relief. "You know where they are."

As long as we were subject to overseas assignments, I wasn't in a position to consider moving Marko from Seattle. When we returned to Washington, D.C., and decided not to take another post abroad, I asked Watson if he thought Marko might want to transfer to a nursing home near me.

He took her to dinner and broached the subject. "I'll pack right away," was her reply. She was eighty-five.

My search for a nursing home in the Washington area was easier because by now I knew what to look for: an attitude of respect, loving care, and professionalism on the part of the nursing staff toward their patients. And Marko craved beauty as well in her surroundings. "It doesn't matter where she is, she won't notice" was the advice of experts who lumped all ageing, deteriorating patients together. Marko noticed.

"What a lovely dining room," she said when I showed her around the Bethesda Nursing Centre. The round tables set for four under sparkling chandeliers, the floor to ceiling windows hung with warm red curtains, a bouquet of yellow and white chrysanthemums on the piano, all pleased her immensely. She needed beautiful surroundings to assure her she was not in a "poor house", a fear from the Great Depression years that still haunted her memory. All the barren, institution-like homes with cold, linoleum floors, hospital green walls, and white iron beds I had quickly eliminated. They were as expensive as the Bethesda Centre where Marko was offered a room in the French Wing with a hospital bed camouflaged in a French Provincial bedstead. We walked down a carpeted hall hung with oil paintings and old prints to see it. Later, Marko told me that she memorised the pictures to find her way to her room.

"Why don't you just try the Bethesda Centre to see how you like it?" suggested Doctor Blake, the shrewd and sympathetic physician I took Marko to. Phrasing it that way, he made the selection of the home Marko's own choice — a crucial factor in any patient's adjustment to a new nursing facility.

"Yes, I think I will try it," Marko decided.

Doctor Blake was in complete agreement with my request to reduce her medications to an absolute minimum. He took her completely off tranquillisers. I felt as if I had won a tremendous victory.

Doctor Blake shook Marko's hand. "I'll come out to Bethesda to visit you soon and see how you're getting along."

Then, walking ahead to the door with me, he said in a low voice, "You know she is going to get much worse and there is nothing we can do about it. There is no treatment that can reverse or arrest dementia. It's a terrible thing to be happening to such a fine woman."

The woman in the room next to Marko's at the Bethesda Nursing Centre had greeted us with the manners of a grande dame. She was dressed in a well-tailored black suit and her hair was freshly set. When she walked on down the hall Marko made a flourish with her hand, pushed up the end of her nose and pursed her lips. "Toffee-nose," she said, but her eyes sparkled with excitement. Here was a woman to watch. No slovenly residents in housecoats and slippers at Bethesda. For the first time in years Marko began to wear her good clothes and comment on what others wore. As a young woman she had taught tailoring and costume designing at the University of Washington. Fabrics, colour and line interested her. As did the decoration of her room. She told me where to put her lamps and pictures, and showed off the room to us and to the women she was making friends with at her dining table, in the lounge and at her poetry class.

"That Russian woman thinks she knows everything about winter. Well, here's a poem I wrote and they printed it!" Marko declared and handed me the Bethesda Centre's newsletter. And there was Marko's poem, as she said, the first of many she wrote that year:

TO WINTER

With bonfires!
Sharp runners on new skates.
And singing in the frosty air.
What could be more fun?

Such a burst of creativity was like a small miracle after the apathy Marko had sunk into at North End. Being off tranquillisers made her much more alert. And the bustle of activities at this new nursing home perked her up beyond all of our expectations. There were birthday parties, skits, sing-alongs, movies, slide talks, book groups, poetry classes, dance groups, even a happy hour — all activities that a patient with dementia could enter into at any level of ability. Marko stayed away from the arts and crafts and went to the dances. "See," she said as she turned slowly around the room for me, "Everyone clapped. I used to love dancing."

She was Mrs Smith again to the nurses and aides, not a small child called Marko. Probably few things wound a person with deteriorating mental ability more than to be treated as a stupid, stubborn child. Condescension breeds resentment and resistance. Slowly much of Marko's resistance evaporated. Her paranoia faded.

"Mrs Smith is so cheerful," the head nurse in the French Wing remarked. "We all enjoy her because she gets so much pleasure out of everything." I was astonished. And my surprise increased when Marko observed how good the food was.

"We try to give the residents variety," the admissions director explained. "Almost all of our patients, however well off they may be, come in here with some degree of malnutrition simply because they long since ceased paying attention to their diet, either due to lack of interest or because of a condition like your mother's where they were unable to care for themselves. The sad thing is that most doctors don't recognise malnutrition in older people.

"Eating can be a major pleasure so we give them a variety of nutritious food and make it look attractive. And we have five meals a day — smaller amounts stretched out over a longer period since it's not comfortable nor good for older people who aren't very active to eat too much at one time."

"It's the life of Riley," Marko told me one morning when I came early and found her sitting up in bed having juice, coffee and a croissant.

I brought her art books, the *National Geographic,* and the *Alaska Magazine,* not because she read any more, (her attention span was too short), but because she liked to look at the pictures. But most important to her was the prestige of having good books and magazines stacked on the shelves of her bookstand. They defined her life. Also for status more than interest she wanted the newspaper delivered to her room by the fresh-faced paper boy who made his daily rounds in the home. All this ritual of her old life strengthened Marko's sense of security and lessened her feelings of abandonment.

My dear old friend, Pat Lax, without being asked,

stopped in regularly on her way home from work. Nothing had to be explained to Pat. She accepted Marko as she was, as did Bill's sister who dropped by with bags of chocolate and bottles of cologne.

Stacy, who was struggling to become an artist, wrote Marko a carefully selected postcard every week with the reproduction of a painting by one of her favourite artists. Marko, proudly showing off the cards, believed that Stacy wrote to her every day. For years she had nurtured Stacy's interest in art. Her belief in her granddaughter's talent had forged a special bond between them.

I spent Wednesday afternoons with Marko and took her home on weekends. When the weather was fine we went to our cabin in the foothills of the Blue Ridge Mountains. A happy routine seemed to be established until one night in February when the head nurse called to tell me that Marko was extremely distraught because she thought I was dead.

The nurse thought if I spoke to her Marko would be reassured and settle down. For twenty minutes or more Marko and I talked on the telephone. Bill spoke to her. Finally she seemed calm, saying, "All right, darling. I know everything is fine now. Good night."

But later that night her delusions returned. Again she was certain I was dead and she had to find me.

The next day the nurse told me how she had tried to reason with her, saying, "Mrs Smith, your daughter is not dead. She is alive and fine. You just talked to her."

But Marko had tossed her head to the side in a defiant little gesture and declared, "Oh, well, I'm not so sure about that. It's just like Luree — always saying everything is all right just to make me feel better. But *I* know she's dead!"

Determined to find me, she ran down the hall and out into the freezing night. Aides rushed to stop her. She beat them off with clenched fists. Eventually they pushed, pulled and persuaded her into a room which they then locked.

"It was a bad night," she told me. "They locked me up and wouldn't let me stay in my own room." She looked very tired.

"But I talked to you on the phone, Marko. You knew I was all right."

"Yes, I must remember that. I try but somehow I can't. I can't remember what I should." She sighed deeply.

But "the incident", as she called it, of the night before was still vivid in her mind. She described her sensations: "I felt wild ... as if I would explode. I went out on to the balcony and tried to climb down. I *had* to do something."

A terrible tension had driven her into a frenzy. Her anxiety was not yet spent. She clutched my hand. "How is Stacy?"

"She's fine, Marko. She's in Boston. Bill and the boys are fine. All of us are all right." I hugged her hard. "Remember, we're fine. We love you. I love you. Remember. Please remember!"

"Yes, I'm trying," she answered softly. "I'm trying all the time. I keep trying to remember."

"If she continues like this we'll have to transfer her to the locked wing. I'm truly sorry," the nurse informed me.

I called Doctor Blake. He prescribed an anti-psychotic drug, Haldol, which is commonly used for dementia. "It's not a tranquilliser," he assured me. "And I'll give her the smallest amount possible." Haldol was supposed to calm Marko's aggressive anxiety, minimise her obsessions, yet not in any way slow her physical reaction. A large claim.

I prayed it would work. I didn't want my mother to be locked up.

# 7

# MESSAGES GARBLED AND CLEAR

> The ability to surprise is a form of independence.
>
> SHIRLEY HAZZARD: *The Transit of Venus*

Death definitely was on Marko's mind. Stacy told us first. She had been to visit Marko by herself and found her looking very serious, sitting in her blue boudoir chair dressed in her gold and orange chiffon dress. "She received me as if she were holding court," Stacy reported. "We chatted about all sorts of things and then I got up to get a glass of water from her bedside table. She stood up and followed me. When I turned around she looked me straight in the eyes and said, quite forcefully, 'What do you think happens when you die?' "

Stacy sank to the edge of the bed, dreading the discussion. Marko sat down next to her, waiting for an answer. Finally Stacy said, "It will be a very warm place filled with light and very beautiful. No one will be afraid."

Marko listened carefully and nodded in agreement, then asked, "Do you think I'll see everyone there? Mama and Papa, Clarence and Tom?"

"Yes," Stacy replied. "It will be a very beautiful place to be."

They sat silently on the edge of the bed for some time. Stacy said there was a very peaceful feeling between them, then she reached out and took Marko's hand and they talked of other things.

A few weeks later on a snowy night Marko looked out of her window and thought she saw Peter Petcoff, our white-haired neighbour, in a coffin covered with snow. She watched and decided that if he wiggled he was still alive. Peter wiggled. Marko slipped her coat on over her nightgown, put on her boots and hat and headed for the door to help him. An aide stopped her. Marko slapped the aide but she didn't fight her. Instead she abandoned her rescue plan and retreated down the hall.

The next day Bill picked Marko up for a birthday party we were having for her and Peter. Marko was sceptical about Peter's coming. When he walked into the living room, she started from her chair, grabbed his hand and said, "How did you get out of your coffin? I couldn't get to you."

Peter, always a gentleman, murmured, "How kind of you."

Also at the birthday party was Marilyn Silverstone, my old friend and colleague, once a Magnum photographer, now a Tibetan-Buddhist nun. With her was a Tibetan lama. Marko was enchanted with the exquisitely mannered, red-robed lama and he with her. He expressed his amazement that she was eighty-six years old, she looked so well.

"You must come again," Marko told the lama. "It would be wonderful if you could lecture to us about Tibet. You would help promote international understanding." The lama gently took Marko's hand and bowed his head respectfully. Marko was very moved.

When I took her back to the nursing home she told the nurses about the lovely party, how Peter got out of his coffin after all, and that the Tibetan lama promised he would come back to lecture about Tibet.

"How nice," the nurses said, nodding their heads.

Some of Marko's references were baffling to me too. More and more it seemed as if she were listening to something inside herself. Her expression was intent but not focused on us. And then, suddenly, she would burst forth with a statement so clear, so exactly like her old self that I could scarcely take it in. This is typical, I later learned, of people suffering from multi-infarct dementia: confusion one moment, then total intellectual capacity the next. The switches are dizzying for those listening.

One of Marko's favourite pastimes was sitting in our kitchen looking out of the glass doors as squirrels played along the garden fence and up and down the pear tree. Once, as I was getting lunch and she was rambling on as usual about the squirrels, laughing from time to time at their antics, she suddenly stopped and said in a loud, clear voice, "Listen, Luree. Listen to me!" I flipped the hamburgers and turned to face her.

"I've had an interesting life," Marko said firmly. "I've done a lot. I've been to a lot of places and I've seen a lot of things. It's been a good life and you must not be sad when I die. I'm ready and I'm not scared. Remember that!" She held me with a steady, loving gaze. Then she pointed out the glass door. "Look! There's another squirrel."

I ran to write down her words as exactly as I could. I knew that until I transcribed them I wouldn't really believe what I heard her say. Once they were in writing I saw that she had given me a talisman, a mantra, a message that I would desperately need for the long way we had yet to travel together.

She had flung this crucial message out like a shipwrecked victim throwing a bottle with a description of her whereabouts into the sea before the rough waves of confusion washed over her again. I was enormously grateful to have caught it.

For some time we had been aware that Marko's hearing loss contributed to her confusion and sense of isolation, but I had done nothing about it because several doctors had advised me that a hearing aid would be of little help to her.

But Marko kept complaining, "What did you say?"

"Why don't you take her to the National Speech and Hearing Testing Centre for an evaluation?" Doctor Blake suggested. His point was so obvious I was ashamed for not seeing it clearly myself. The point is that just because a person is suffering from dementia does not mean one should stop listening to her complaints and dismiss them as delusions or as inevitable infirmities of age, unimportant or unsolvable.

A loss of hearing, so common in old age, can be a powerful cause of depression. When a person sees the lips of others moving, but hears no sound, it is frightening. She is isolated, watching the world like a silent film with everybody else tuned into the sound, nodding and laughing at lines she does not hear. Small wonder that hearing loss fosters suspicion and paranoia.

Marko was very pleased to take the hearing test. She sat in a sound-proof room with headphones on. I watched her from the control room where the audiologist spoke into a microphone and sent Marko special sounds from a panel large and sophisticated enough to fly Concorde.

We knew that she had a hearing loss in simple terms of volume — about a 40 per cent loss, the audiologist said, which was in the range of good for her age. But it was in the area of hearing acuity that she suffered most. This loss of hearing means a narrowing of the frequency range in which one receives sounds. Consonants are in the high frequency range and vowels in the low. Her range had narrowed, as it does for most older people. This meant her ability to distinguish sounds was impaired. And her impaired hearing was further complicated by her TIAs. What she did hear was muddled and would get worse.

As the audiologist said words and phrases to Marko through the earphones, she asked Marko to repeat them back to her. "Crust," said the audiologist. "Curusoe," said Marko. A hearing mistake understandable to me. But when the audiologist said "red" and Marko repeated "bark", her hearing distortion was dramatised so that I understood as I never had before one of the reasons why our communication was becoming so difficult.

For half an hour Marko happily repeated totally different words and phrases from those spoken by the audiologist. They made no sense whatever to me, but the audiologist found a clear, predictable pattern of hearing acuity loss. That accounted for many of Marko's bizarre statements. She was receiving distorted messages.

"Remember," the audiologist warned me, "it does no good at all to shout the same words at her when you think she has not heard you correctly. She may not have heard you in terms of volume, but more likely she has not been able to distinguish the words you said. You must rephrase and use different words entirely until you think she understands what you are saying."

A hard lesson to learn. Much easier to shout.

Marko also had difficulty understanding conversation when background noises were present. This, too, is a common problem among older people suffering from a gradual deterioration of hearing: the brain becomes less efficient in the complex process of interpreting signals and discriminating between wanted and unwanted sounds. Sorting out sounds in a noisy room is a taxing process under the best of conditions and Marko's dementia compounded her problem.

Still, she wanted a hearing aid. She had been so insistent that she was physically fit that I appreciated how keenly she felt her hearing problem was cutting her off from us when she asked the audiologist if she could try the hearing aid. Patiently the audiologist explained to Marko that a hearing aid would amplify sounds that she had become used to not hearing at all — that it did not make just the soft sounds she wanted to hear louder — and that with her particular problem she probably would be unable to tolerate loud sounds. To demonstrate she fitted an aid into Marko's ear, then slowly opened the door of the testing room. The door squeaked. Marko jumped out of her chair, tearing the aid from her ear. She never asked for one again.

But the testing process was beneficial to both of us in ways I had not anticipated. Marko and I learned that hearing loss is not a simple problem of volume. It was apparent now why Marko was uninterested in TV: she couldn't hear it clearly no matter how much we increased the volume and there was only one chance for her to catch what the speakers said. Our family, on the other hand, became adept at multiple phrase-making. We rephrased rather than shouted. And our messages got through more often.

Next Marko decided her teeth were falling out. I pointed out that she had splendid teeth, they were the envy of Watson and me: she had two small fillings and one gold crown. But, remembering our new policy of paying attention to all of her complaints, however wild, I bundled her off to the dentist.

"Marvellous," said Doctor Baxter, tapping with his pick the tiny gold filling in her front tooth. "You see this filling? It's at least sixty years old. It was hammered in fleck by fleck. They only did that years ago in the West."

Marko beamed. "I had to have it done in White

Bird, Idaho, the first year I taught there." Quickly I calculated that would have been in about 1912.

"Wonderful work. We can't afford to do that any more. You're very lucky. Splendid teeth." Doctor Baxter smiled at her. "But she has such heavy tartar deposits they're causing her gums to recede badly," he said to me, raising his eyebrows in reproach. "She's suffering quite a lot of discomfort."

Score another point for paying attention. There was a basis for Marko's hyperbole. The tartar deposits that were causing all of her teeth to ache could have led to her losing them. Her saying they were falling out was not far wrong.

Marko was waiting in the lobby the next time I went to pick her up from the nursing home. For a moment I didn't recognise her. She had cut her long hair and had a permanent wave. "We begged her not to do it," the young physiotherapist ran up to tell me. "Nobody grows hair like that any more. It was beautiful."

Marko's eyes sparkled. She grinned at my shocked expression. A little group of nurses and aides gathered around us, recounting their protestations and Marko's determination to have her hair cut and her insistence that they not call me for permission. "Before I made her appointment with the beauty shop I said, 'Mrs Smith, are you absolutely sure you want to do this?' " the head nurse reported. Marko shook her head enthusiastically. That was how it had happened. She had staged her little event to perfection and played it out with relish.

When I brought her home Bill was stunned. "My God, Marko! What have you done with your hair?"

"Cut it to surprise you." Marko laughed with delight.

Scott gasped. "I can't believe it. You look so different. Nice. But different."

"Why did you do it?" Bill asked.

"To get attention, of course," Marko shot back. "I don't know now what I can do next. I may have to cut off my big toe."

At the time I think we half believed she might do it. But she was slipping fast beyond the point where she could will her actions. If I visited her in late afternoon her confusion was marked — the 'Sundown Syndrome', Doctor Blake called it — an increased disorientation resulting from a loss of visual clarity as dusk settles in. This and an 'early morning confusion' before she shook off sleep are common states with many older people and intensified for those with dementia.

Extreme patience was needed. Marko seemed to be living a slow-motion life. Trying to hurry her was useless. It only increased her confusion. And that summer I was in a hurry, in a panic, under the pressure of a September deadline to finish writing my book.

Marko's pace of life and mine couldn't have been more incompatible.

When Watson and I had finally accepted the fact that Marko was slipping into dementia and we made the excruciating decision to put her in a nursing home, it was with the knowledge that neither of us could have cared for her with the patience and skill that nursing care professionals could provide. Now, more than ever, I was grateful we had made that decision in spite of the criticism we received from well-meaning but, to my mind, unthinking friends. We couldn't completely shake our guilt, so strong is society's general condemnation of nursing homes, but we had learned to live with it. Much of the censure of nursing care is justified; inspection and exposure of substandard nursing homes is essential. But let us not forget to praise those which are well-run shelters for brain-damaged people whose families cannot provide constant care.

Constant care, even with outside help, calls for saintly patience. Martyrs do best in this role. I am neither a saint nor a martyr. Much as I loved Marko, had she lived with me we would have destroyed each other. As it was, she lived in a setting geared to her pace of life. Instead of sitting morosely in the empty daytime quiet of my house with a hired caretaker to watch her while I was out, she was in a stimulating environment with a wide range of people and activities to ward off lethargy and depression. A dietitian prepared her meals, a physiotherapist coaxed her through her exercises, and a beauty operator washed and set her hair.

Had Marko been with me all of the time I couldn't have coped. One afternoon just as I was ready to take her back to the home, she inadvertently locked herself in the bathroom. The door had an old-fashioned pushbutton lock in the door knob which, once pushed in, had to be turned to the left sharply before turning it to the right to open the door. I cursed myself for not having changed the knob to avert such a predicament.

"Turn the handle to the left, Marko," I shouted through the door, knowing the situation was hopeless. I wanted to scream. But it would have rattled her completely. I tried to calculate how long it would take the fire department to come and get her out. Could I get her through the rush-hour traffic back to the home, meet my colleague at the plane as planned, and make it to the evening class I was teaching?

"It's all right, Marko," I called in a smothered voice. "Just keep turning the door knob. It will open."

Miraculously it did. Like the teacher who would gladly sever the head of the dawdling, day-dreaming child but is able to restrain herself only because she can send him home at two o'clock, I was able to curb my impatience with Marko because our time together was limited. Short-term patience I could manage.

In the country I was less irritated with her slowness. Like a small child she had to be reminded to wipe her bottom and pull up her pants after she went to the toilet and to be watched constantly so she wouldn't wander out into the street. At our mountain cabin it didn't matter. The tangles of honeysuckles and pine forest stopped her from roaming too far. And there she was more at peace, less inclined to become agitated. No phone rang, people weren't rushing in and out. It was blissfully quiet. She sat on the deck stroking our Siamese cat curled in her lap and watched the cows graze slowly up a distant hill. I gave her a broad-brimmed picture hat I had worn to the Queen's Garden Party in London to shade her eyes and when I brought her a cup of tea she curled her little finger affectedly as she took the cup and mimicking an English accent said, "I do thank you, my dear."

We hauled a heavy duty washing machine up to the cabin because she was becoming increasingly incontinent. The aides had tried taking her to the bathroom to empty her bladder at regular intervals but she so resented being told what to do that she refused to cooperate. That stubborn will of hers kept her fighting off any interference with her independence.

In the early spring we had given up taking her to restaurants for fear of an "accident" and switched to picnicking in Rock Creek Park where a puddle on a picnic bench could easily be sluiced off with water from the creek. Eventually the head nurse convinced me that putting nappies on her was the only answer. To ask my fastidious mother to accept nappies I thought would mortify her. A measure of how far she had slipped was that she scarcely objected. "I wonder when I'll get over this," she said as I pinned the bulky nappy around her waist.

"Nothing is wrong with her sphincter muscles," Doctor Blake explained. It was not a muscular problem, but a mental one. Such irony! Here she was with an excellent body: all vital organs working well, fine colouring, not one varicose vein, excellent appetite, only the control centre was defective.

Bad enough to have a child wet the bed, but when an adult does there is a flood. I set my alarm for 2 a.m. to get Marko up in hopes I could get her to the toilet in time. But when I tried to awaken her she fought me like a tiger.

That summer she lost all ability to dress herself. She put one dress on top of another and she could no longer take her own bath. Leaning over the bathtub I scrubbed her smooth back and reminded her how Virgil used to say she had the prettiest little ass he ever saw. Marko giggled and made a face pretending to be shocked by my speech. Then one day another clogging of her communication system cut off another simple motor function. She couldn't understand how to get up and step out of the bathtub. I put one of her hands on the bathtub ledge, the other around the handle above the soap dish and encouraged her to pull herself up. She looked at me helplessly and sat there. No amount of cajoling or demonstrating how she should pull herself to her feet stimulated any effort on her part. She could not initiate the proper movement. She couldn't even try. She could not conceive what trying meant. Finally I took off my shoes, climbed in the tub behind her, braced my feet on the rubber non-slip pads, and squatted down to put both arms around her. Praying we wouldn't crash on the hard enamel of the tub, I heaved her up. She laughed, bewildered. After that we gave up the bubble baths she loved and I scrubbed her down in the shower.

Her walk became more markedly a shuffle, an abnormality associated with multi-infarct dementia. At the cabin she shuffled from the deck to the porch. "I'm lost," she cried.

Once she came and stood by the kitchen table where I was writing. Impulsively she grabbed my hand to kiss it and press it to her cheek. "When I know where I am it is all right," she said softly. "I'm happy."

Ellen sent Marko's mother-of-pearl opera glasses for her to use bird-watching at the cabin and in her room at Bethesda Nursing. There was a cherry tree directly outside her window. For hours she sat contentedly watching the birds flutter up and down the branches picking at the hard little red cherries. She dozed over our photograph albums that she once loved to look at, remembering our trips together and the wonderful years when she and Virgil were in Lahore, Pakistan, and we were in Dhaka, Bangladesh, when Stacy, Scott and Blair were wide-eyed youngsters flying back and forth the thousand miles between us. But the photographs jogged her memory less and less.

I felt there still was so much to say, so many questions to ask her if only I could catch her in those narrowing slits of time when her mind was clear. She had more of those moments at the cabin so I gave up writing on weekends and asked for an extension of the deadline on my book.

Autumn came and somehow, by October, I finished my book and was ready to go to London for the final editorial work. Bill planned to join me after my work was done so that we could have a short holiday visiting an old friend in Portugal.

"I hate to leave Marko. It seems as if she has so little time left," I told Scott. By now he was working in Washington and living a few blocks from us on Capitol Hill.

"Don't worry. I'll take her out," he comforted me.

Marko understood that at last my book was finished and I had to go. "I've always told you, finish what you start," she said. It was true. She had.

After we were gone, Scott visited Marko and shortly before we returned planned a gala day for her at the National Gallery of Art. He drove her through Rock Creek Park, the winding, woodsy route she loved so well. Along the way she always pointed out the shapes of trees and stones or the way a log had fallen across the creek. With her sharp eyes she saw squirrels and an occasional raccoon before we ever did.

Scott stopped the car on the circular drive in front of the Gallery, helped her shuffle to a wheelchair in the lobby and told her to wait while he parked. Then he wheeled her through the spacious galleries where her favourite Impressionist paintings hung. Sharing her preferences (for she had helped train his eye) he held her chair longest in front of the Manets, Renoirs, Cassats, Monets and Matisses she loved best. Joyously Marko called them by name, her reliable old friends she had lived with so long. Their exquisite colours and wonderful light had refuelled her romantic dreams. And she was a powerful dreamer. On moonlight nights when I was a child, she would lean out of my bedroom window gazing at the moon's shadows on the lawn, telling me how filled with beauty the world was if only one learned to look. "Look!" she exhorted Stacy, Blair and Scott. "It is what *you* see, not what others tell you." Her dreams empowered me. Now she struggled to pass them on to her grandchildren — her future, her immortality.

"So beautiful, so peaceful. I love the Impressionists," Marko declared to Scott.

"So do I." He kissed her cheek.

Then he wheeled her into the solarium so she could see the tiers of russett and yellow chrysanthemums circling the fountain and massed under the great green fronds of tropical plants. She rubbed a thick green leaf between her fingers and smiled at him. Since it was such a fine sunny October day they sat in the car awhile watching some rosy-cheeked children playing tag on the Mall.

"I love children," she said. "A marvellous day, Scott. So beautiful."

He drove her back through Rock Creek Park. She was very tired but happy.

"We'll do it again, Marko," Scott promised.

"Wonderful," she agreed. But that was her last outing.

# 8

# ONE TOUGH LADY

It is in the hospital, of all places, that the difference between the desires of the physician and the desires of the patients clash hardest.

ERIC HODGKINS: *Episode: An Accident in My Skull*

The telephone rang, shrill and insistent. I shot out of bed like a bullet from the dark barrel of a rifle and landed on my target. Then I woke. The phone was quiet. The whole house was quiet. Bill, still warm in bed, was breathing regularly, heavily. The ringing was in my dream; it didn't have to be answered. I already knew what the call was for: to inform me that my mother was dead.

For the last year every ring of the phone had promised me that message. I pulled up the window blind. The street lamp, a ball of pale yellow light, was burning under the bare, dark branches of the sycamore tree. Marko had invaded my dreams. I slept lightly, as I had when my children were small, waiting for the call, wanting to be there in time to hold her hand and comfort her.

At 8.30 am the call came. The head nurse on duty at the nursing home told me Marko "appeared to have had a stroke". After she had eaten a croissant and drunk a cup of coffee, she slowly tumbled from a sitting position off the side of her bed. Two aides in the hall saw her as she slowly fell. They were not able to reach her in time but it was a soft fall. She did not bruise or hurt herself. When Bill and I arrived there was a tall green oxygen cylinder beside her bed. She was hooked to it by a tube and a plastic mask over her nose. I kissed her, cradling her hand, and called to her.

"A stroke is an easy way to go," a nurse said, smiling sympathetically at us.

Suddenly Marko had a large spasm. Her face flushed red, her left leg jack-knifed. Another explosion in her brain like the one that had tumbled her off the bed. A real stroke, not a transient ischemic attack. All of those little TIAs were preludes to this grand finale. Her eyes opened wide and I desperately wanted her to live. Then her eyes shut and she was gone again.

"Mrs Smith, you have had a stroke. Your doctor is coming to see you." The nurse leaned close to her, repeating this information in a calm, clear voice. Then she asked, "Are you warm enough?"

"Very warm," Marko mumbled.

She hadn't spoken before. "We assume all stroke patients can hear us," the nurse explained. "And we tell them what is happening so they won't be frightened." Marko had had a haemorrhage or blood clot on the right side of her brain. Consequently her left side was paralysed.

"Marko, do you know we're here with you? That Bill and I are here?"

"Yes, darling," came her muffled reply. Tears of relief flooded my eyes; I had reached her in time!

She had another spasm, painful to watch. Alternately Bill and I talked to her, stroked her hand and kissed her forehead. Doctor Blake was out of town, as one's own doctor always seems to be in times of crises. His substitute was on call to come. Four hours passed. But Marko was not an emergency. She could wait. Still, Bill went to phone the doctor's office again.

Another spasm began. I clasped Marko's good right hand. Instead she passed a volley of gas like the roll of drums. It was so startling I laughed. Feigning shock I said, "Well, Mrs Smith, I certainly hope you feel better!"

Unmoving, eyes closed, Marko answered softly, "I do."

Mrs Neal from across the hall peered anxiously into Marko's room to inquire about "my friend". A physiotherapist dropped by to say, "I'll miss Mrs

Smith. She never complained. She was cheerful and liked to joke." "Well, she *is* very sweet," remarked Bunny, one of Marko's favourite aides. "But boy, sometimes when she's not, she's something from the zoo."

At 2.24 pm Dr Howe came, a kindly man with grey hair and a quiet air of competence. "It's a moderate stroke, although it will be twenty-four to forty-eight hours before we know if the period of strokes is over," he told us. "And she is *eighty-six*."

I was ready with my prepared reply: "We understand. Please do not make any heroic efforts to keep her alive. She's lived a good long life and she would hate to be further impaired. Just do what is necessary to keep her as comfortable as you possibly can." I had rehearsed this set speech hundreds of times so that I could say it convincingly when I knew my heart would be in ascendance, holding on to life under any terms. By her own example, I was certain that Marko would choose non-treatment for herself as she had for Virgil when he had his stroke. "He would hate to come back half himself," she had said then. And he was lucky. He did not have to. His stroke was fatal.

The prospect of Marko recovering to some sort of semi-vegetable state and being moved into the skilled care section of the nursing home was too distressing to contemplate. I had walked through that wing and seen the patients strapped to their chairs, twitching, moaning, drooling, some reaching out to clutch at me as I walked by, others calling, "Help me, help me!" A collection of ancient horrors I could not bear to see again.

"Marko," I said silently as I stood by her bed holding her hand, waiting for the ambulance to come. "Please die now. Please go quickly like Virgil." But my treacherous heart held on to her. It ached with the impossible wish that she would live, that she would recover even to the same demented state that she had been in before the stroke when for brief flashes she was her rational self and we made contact. Our bond of love was too old, too strong, twisted with too many knots to easily loosen. But I tried. "Marko, let go," I whispered in her ear. "It's all right. You can go now. We love you. Everything is all right. Be peaceful. Have a good journey. Goodbye, Marko. Goodbye." I smoothed her forehead and kissed her soft cheeks. She looked serene.

Bunny came in again. "Most of her clothes won't be any good for her when she comes back. You'll have to think about getting her gowns that open all the way down the front."

"Comes back?" I echoed.

"Oh sure," Bunny grinned. "She'll be back. We know all about that. She's a fighter. You can tell which ones will give up when something hits them. They just die. Others put up a good fight to live. That's your mother. She'll fight. She's one tough lady. She'll be back here. You just wait and see."

Suddenly I felt very tired and confused. I let go of Marko's hand and sat down. Bill came back with coffee. We counted the number of seizures Marko had: five in all, and compared their intensities. Never having witnessed any strokes before, they seemed to us severe. "Will she live through all of those?" I asked Bill. He shook his head, not knowing.

I packed a small bag with her toothbrush, comb, nail file, baby powder, hand lotion and one robe that opened all the way down the front. A nurse checked in and suggested I remove Marko's gold bracelet, the one Ellen sent her which she wore all the time. "I'm going to take your bracelet off, Marko. I'll keep it while you're in hospital. Is that all right with you?"

"Yes," she answered softly.

Eyes still closed, wrapped in a blanket like a mummy, Marko was slipped on to the stretcher and into the ambulance by the driver and medic. I sat beside her. Bill followed in our car. I had persuaded the driver not to use the siren. Quietly we wound our way through Rock Creek Park. I described to Marko the familiar landmarks we were passing: the arched bridge, Miller's cabin, the Old Stone Mill, and how the autumn leaves blazed crimson and yellow. "Squeeze my hand if you can hear me," I said. Weakly she squeezed back and murmured, "Colours are lovely."

Exiting from the park, we turned on to Pennsylvania Avenue and pulled into the emergency entrance of George Washington University Hospital, the hospital famous for its trauma unit, a teaching hospital with skilled doctors, superb emergency care and the latest technology. Quickly Marko was checked in and assigned a room. Bill and I followed as she was wheeled down the hall. A brisk woman doctor came in and examined her briefly. She asked us to wait for the intern who would take Marko's medical history. Clipboard in hand he arrived a few minutes later, tousle-haired in casual cords and a plaid shirt, ivy-league brightness, smiling at me confidently. I had a flash of foreboding. Immediately he recommended a neurologist be called in to confirm Marko's diagnosis. "Please, no!" I cut in. "Don't put her through any unnecessary tests. Doctor Howe said she has suffered several strokes. The nurses witnessed them. They've seen lots of strokes. There's no question of what happened to her," I pleaded.

"She needs a CAT scan," the intern answered.

I knew that a CAT scan was a highly sophisticated diagnostic tool. It can locate the precise spot of a blood clot or haemorrhage in the skull by x-rays which feed signals into a high speed computer. With younger, stronger people the results of a CAT scan sometimes indicate delicate brain surgery.

"But given her age and medical history, what would

you do with my mother if you did discover the site of her clot or haemorrhage?" I asked the doctor.

"Nothing," she acceded.

I could see her struggling with the need to allow the intern to follow a standard procedure for stroke victims and thus gain essential experience. Against this she weighed my plea for Marko's peace and comfort on the basis of her age and condition. "Why," I asked myself, "did I ever let Marko come to a teaching hospital?" That fine balance between the patient's needs and the need for the doctors to gain more knowledge and experience surely is tipped in their favour here.

I stared hard at the doctor. I could see her waiver. Finally she vetoed the neurologist and the CAT scan. But she did agree with the intern that Marko should have a chest x-ray to check for fluid in her lungs. I remember Doctor Blake saying the previous winter when Marko had a chest cold that pneumonia used to be called the old people's friend because it let them die peacefully, but now we insisted on medications to cure pneumonia and let them live a little longer to die from something more cruel and devastating.

"Let's step outside," the doctor said, glancing at Marko's still form on the bed. With a sudden pang of guilt I wondered if Marko had heard our arguments. Surely she had.

Outside the door I asked the doctor what she

thought Marko's chances were. She declined to make a prognosis, saying instead that in the cases of strokes one never knew, and she left for her next case. Bill went out to repark the car. I sat in an alcove across from Marko's room while the intern asked me questions and filled in the pages of his clipboard. Trolleys with patients encased in white were trundled up and down the hall. Nurses bustled by. The fast pace of this first-class hospital increased my apprehension. Once again I explained to the intern: absolutely no extraordinary measures to keep Marko alive.

"It's hard to die in a hospital," he agreed, but he spoke perfunctorily, from a frame of reference totally different from mine. I knew he lived in a different world, a sick world, where there was only one goal: to keep patients alive and help them get well. A commendable goal, of course, but a narrow one. Narrow like his high-technology medical life that allows young medical students no time for reading or space for the kind of broad experience that develops wisdom and compassion. He was hard and bright. A highly skilled technician.

Marko should not be here at all, I realised. A hospital is no place for an elderly patient close to death. She could have been cared for more tenderly in the nursing home. But the rationale for bringing her here was economic: unless she were in a hospital she would not be eligible for Medicare to cover her doctors' fees and possible convalescence costs. And it was a reflex action to head for the hospital in the event of a physical crisis.

Marko's medical history taken, we went across the hall to her room. A huge x-ray machine on wheels stood outside her door. Marko's bed was still rolled up and there she lay as the x-ray technician had left her, uncovered, turned awkwardly on her left side, head back, gown askew, right breast and shoulder bare, a twisted, forlorn figure like someone dead and washed ashore. I was furious.

"No more tests! Promise me that!" I turned on the intern. "Your supervising doctor agreed."

"Okay. Okay." He put his pencil on his ear and left. A dull and pointless case for him. My impulse was to scoop Marko up off the hard hospital bed and take her home. Take her away from this efficient, sterile atmosphere, to let her die lying on soft pillows soothed by soft voices, with our Siamese cat she loved curled at her feet. But I didn't know how. I had no experience with death. We had handed Virgil over to the doctors and now I had done the same with Marko.

Bill came back. It took both of us to lift her dead weight into a comfortable position. We put her hospital gown back on and pulled the blanket up over her. I clasped her hand and asked her to squeeze mine if she could hear me. Very faintly I felt the press of her fingers against mine.

"Are you comfortable now? Are you warm enough? Do you want me to stay with you a while?" I asked anxiously. But no sound came from her. She could no longer answer me.

Then Bill put his arm around my shoulders and gently steered me towards the door.

# 9

# THE EIGHTH DAY

> I shall be like that tree. I shall die first at the top.
>
> JONATHAN SWIFT

The hospital seemed eerily quiet the day after Marko's stroke. It was Sunday. Scott and I walked down the empty corridor and turned the corner. There at the nurses' station was the same intern I had argued with the night before. "Oh, hi," he said. Instantly I knew. The look in his eyes and the defensive hunch of his shoulders told me that he had put Marko through a CAT scan after all. "I tried to call you," he protested. "Anyway, the results did not indicate treatment. I hope you're not angry." It was too late for anger. All I felt was a depressing sense of powerlessness. There was no way I could protect Marko here in hospital. I wondered if she had been handled roughly like last night when they gave her a chest x-ray or gently, by different technicians with some sensitivity for the fragility of her age. Scott opened the door to her room.

A nurse's aide, struggling to put a clean sheet under Marko's recumbent body, looked up and asked me to help hold Marko when she rolled her on her side to slip the sheet under her. "We're short-handed this weekend and it really takes two people to move a patient like this," she apologised. "I just can't manage it alone."

Marko's left forearm was splinted with the needle of her IV tube taped on to the back of her hand. She was receiving glucose and water intravenously but no more oxygen tubes were inserted into her nose. Great black and blue bruises covered the back of her right hand where numerous blood samples had been taken. The needle pricks were still visible like tattoo marks made by a beginner without a design. Her eyes were closed. She was breathing heavily.

"It's me," Scott said, bending down to kiss her. She pressed his hand and mumbled something we could not catch. Still, it was encouraging. Her eyelids twitched but did not open. She lay partially paralysed, unmoving.

Scott reminded her of their visit to the National Gallery just the Sunday before. "Do you remember the Renoirs and the Gauguins, Marko?"

"Yes," came the faint reply. Scott and I glanced at each other hopefully. "You liked the 'Girl with the Watering Can'," he encouraged her. "Remember, Marko? Remember the big Renoir?"

"The children — lovely." Her answer was faint but distinct. Eagerly he continued to recount their last day together. Her breathing was so heavy she was almost gasping. But she began to punctuate Scott's account with a "yes", or a "lovely". Once she said, "Beautiful, just beautiful," and Scott and I smiled at each other across her bed. When we told her we were leaving but would be back soon Marko blurted out a full sentence: "It was good of you to come by." Such a statement from her semi-conscious form seemed miraculous. And in the presence of a seeming miracle one hopes against all reason and previous knowledge for a stunning resurrection. We left buoyed with the hope that she would recover.

But recovery for a stroke victim is seldom complete. Perhaps thirty per cent are able to make a good recovery. The other seventy per cent are partially or totally handicapped. They have been wounded and mauled and will never be the complete person they were before. The older they are, the less hope that the brain can accommodate and compensate for the blown-out areas. And Marko's little strokes, her TIAs, already had done permanent damage to portions of her brain. I dreaded the possibility that these major strokes coupled with her TIAs would leave her able only to vegetate with a few rudimentary reflexes working: paralysed on one side, immobile, mute and uncomprehending — a state I knew she had desperately feared.

"It's time to die, Marko," I told her the next day. She squeezed my hand.

By the third day she was completely unconscious. "Comatose," the nurse said. "She doesn't respond to pain stimulus."

"It means she is completely comfortable. She's not suffering," Doctor Howe comforted me. "It's like an anaesthesia or a deep sleep." Her prognosis now was serious. There was irregularity in her breathing. Her pulse was slow. Doctor Howe advised me to give up her room in the nursing home.

"Really, a stroke is the best way to go. No pain," Watson said on the telephone from Seattle. We agreed not to have a memorial service right away. We needed a little time to think about it. Marko had told me that she wanted to be cremated with her ashes scattered over the waters of Puget Sound. It was romantic, unconventional. I wasn't quite sure how to do it. "Don't worry now," Watson counselled. "There's no hurry."

First there was her room at the nursing home to be cleared out. A few boxes of books, some pictures, lamps and small tables, armloads of clothes and two boudoir chairs. I carted them to the station wagon. So final, so quick. A maintenance man came to take down her name plate outside the door. In a brief afternoon all traces of Mrs Margaret Watson Smith were gone. Her cosy little room with the blue flowered wallpaper was bare.

On the fourth day a sign saying Seizure Precautions was placed on the hospital wall above the head of Marko's bed. Next to it was taped a padded tongue depressant. A light on the panel above her bed illuminated Priority. The IV bottle dripped Dextrose, saline and potassium at the rate of nineteen drops a minute into the thin plastic tube attached to the needle taped into her swollen right hand.

A sympathetic young nurse came in to give Marko a bath. She asked me to help her roll Marko over and dry and powder her. Then I rubbed her legs and feet with hand lotion. The nurse showed me how to roll a pink foam rubber mouth cleaner around Marko's teeth and gums. "You know it helps you a lot to do things like this," she said "Why don't you brush her hair too?"

"When my mother dies and is cremated, what happens to her wedding ring?" I asked the nurse.

"They cut it off at the funeral home. Why don't you take it off now?"

I couldn't answer. It would be the final stripping of the body. The thick gold band she had worn night and day for sixty-two years, caking its gleaming surface with soap and clay and paint and garden earth.

With an encouraging smile the nurse handed me a small plastic bowl of water, a bar of yellow soap and a white wash-cloth and towel. "Today her IV is in her right hand. Tomorrow it will be in her left," she reminded me.

Feeling ghoulish and uneasy, I picked up Marko's hand and stroked it. Her fingers were very swollen. Gently I placed her hand in the bowl of warm water, lathered it with soap and worked the wedding ring off her fourth finger. "I'll keep it for Stacy," I told her, and patted her hand dry. She lay so terribly still, rigid on her paralysed left side, limp on her right. Her face was slightly puffed, smoothing out the wrinkles, making her look serene and beautiful. I brushed her hair and talked to her about the things we had done this last year — our family gatherings, our picnics, the Easter concert at the National Cathedral when she had looked delightedly around at the huge audience and declared, "What a wonderful opportunity to study profiles!", our trips to our mountain cabin, the way she loved to ride in the car with Bill when he was doing errands, Clio purring in her lap. There was no way to know if she heard me. She was comatose, no longer able to squeeze my hand. But I had to say these things. I wanted to fill her mind with pleasant memories, to push out whatever dreads or fears, old hurts or hates that might be crowding forward. I wanted her to stay serene, to go in peace. There was so much to say. But after an hour or so I left, exhausted, and took the Metro home. Once inside the door, the knot burgeoning in my chest burst out in a high shrill wail. Clio flew up the stairs in terror. I paced through the house sobbing and shouting curses at the fates that had felled Marko and savaged her body, cheating her of a swift, clean death.

Unable to do anything more for her, it was almost a relief and certainly a distraction to start planning her memorial service.

"How can we mark her death?" I asked Jane Weld. Jane had been my ballast through the long passage with Marko. Her home just off Rock Creek Park was my safe haven when I could scarcely weather the anguish of watching Marko deteriorate.

"Whatever you do," Jane advised, "remember that the memorial service is not important for *her.* It's for the living. You don't want a minister who never knew her trying to talk about her life. Marko might rise up and smite him. She lived life well. A service is not important for her. Whatever you decide to do, it won't be any good to go through with something which would not have happy associations for her. I'm sure your children would agree."

She was right, they did. "The important thing is that we were all together in August," Blair called from Seattle. "Marko really enjoyed it. Don't worry about a memorial service."

"Think how brave she was to make a major move when she was eighty-five," Stacy phoned from Boston. "She always wanted to be in the swing of things. Try to look at it this way. Marko's making it a little easier for us by going slowly. She's giving us time to say 'goodbye'. Not like Virgil. He went too quickly. It was too much of a shock. Instead she's giving us time to adjust and say our last farewells."

The next day I waited until just before I had to teach my evening class to visit Marko. The Seizure Precautions sign above her bed was gone. Her Priority light was not on. Eyes closed, she looked peaceful. Her breathing was slow and regular. Sitting beside her bed, holding her hand, I wished fervently that she would finally slip away.

"Let go, Marko," I pleaded. "Please. It's time. Try to let go." But I knew that her tenacity was a deep habit. She had fought through too many crises, defied the fates and come through too often to give up easily. In the mountains of Idaho she had helped her mother treat rattlesnake bites, gunshot wounds, and barbed wire infections. In those days before penicillin, when his appendix ruptured, she had stayed nursing Virgil after a doctor had said he was gone. For four nights she had kept me, an infant of eight months, upright on her lap when whooping cough threatened my life. These were her triumphs against death, the stories of victory that she chose to remember and pass on to me. All of her instincts, all of her experience forged her defiant hold on to life. So how could she let go now?

Suddenly her fingers pressed against my palm. A chill ran through me. "Marko," I called, leaning close to her. "Squeeze my hand if you can hear me." Hardly breathing, I waited. No response. I stroked her forehead, smoothed her eyebrows and called again. Still no response. She must have had a small, involuntary spasm.

"Your mother seems to have levelled off," Doctor Howe said on the seventh day. "Her blood pressure and pulse are normal. In fact," he added, "she's less unconscious than before — that is, she is a bit closer to consciousness. Still, there is no significant, measurable improvement."

On the eighth day the first thing Bill and I noticed when we walked into Marko's hospital room was that her IV bottle was gone. Then we saw that her great brown eyes were open looking straight at us.

# 10

# A Good Mother

> She fought against all of her ills with amazing elasticity, forgot them, baffled them, inflicted on them signal if temporary defeats ...
>
> COLETTE: *My Mother's House*

Fourteen days after her massive stroke Marko was sitting in a chair, tied to its back by a wide harness so she would not fall out. To see her sitting up being examined by an intern was a terrific shock. I had mourned her expected death and begun to plan her funeral service. But the fact is that strokes maim more often than they kill. A portion of the victim's brain is destroyed by a sudden cut-off of the blood supply of oxygen. This cut-off is due to an occlusion in a blood vessel in the neck or the brain. It may be caused by a blood clot lodged in the blood vessel, which is called a thrombosis. Or it may be the result of an aneurysm, which is a localised dilation of a blood vessel that fills with fluid or clotted blood to form a pulsating tumour blocking the normal blood supply. Or the stroke victim may have suffered a cerebral haemorrhage when a blood vessel in the brain bursts, causing bleeding into the brain tissue or spaces surrounding the brain.

Whatever the cause, a thrombosis, an aneurysm, or a cerebral haemorrhage, a completed stroke, unlike a TIA, always leaves the victim with some degree of impairment. Residua, the doctors call it. But they seldom know exactly what or how much the resulting impairment will be. Until the anatomy and functions of the brain are better mapped and understood, it is impossible to know precisely which area controls what functions, although scientific studies have demonstrated that specific skills are lodged in either the right or the left hemispheres of the brain. The two halves of the brain, with their billions of nerve cells, are connected by the crossover of a myriad of nerve pathways, so that if a stroke occurs any place in the right side of the brain the victim will be affected somewhere on the left side of her body and vice versa. That was where Marko was hit. In her right brain hemisphere. Her cerebrovascular accident, as strokes are medically termed, made her left side paralysed, her left arm and leg useless.

The right hemisphere of the brain where her accident occurred is the source of a person's sense of space, orientation, proportion and perspective. Hence it is considered to be the artistic side of the brain, the intuitive and creative, the seat of non-verbal mental activity. It is the side of the brain that seems to give us our subtlety and intuitive perceptions, our creative powers. If true, what was left of the artist in Marko was irrevocably gone.

What was undamaged (except spottily by her previous TIAs) was the logical left hemisphere where language and language-related skills reside. Over the next few weeks Marko slowly regained her speech. In that she was lucky. The loss of speech by stroke victims whose accidents occur in their left brain hemisphere is termed aphasia, surely one of the most agonising of all stroke impairments. But her speech was intact and I was talking to the left hemisphere of her brain, to the side that is called dominant because it seems to control our sense of logic and our rational and analytical thought. And for right-handed people, the left side of the brain controls their right, writing hand.

But Marko was diminished by more than half because if it is true that originality and creativity spring from the other side of the brain, then for her, like most artists, the right brain hemisphere was her more highly developed half. Doctors have observed that patients with right hemisphere injuries seem to be robbed of an emotional quality. Functioning mainly with the logical left, they are known in clinical studies for their amusing "one-liners" — their grammar is fine but their feelings are limited. "May I use your bathroom?" I asked Marko many weeks later. "I'll be quick."

"Of course, my dear, but I'd rather you be careful than quick," she shot back — a quip not unlike the old, integrated Marko, but no arched look or laughter followed. She just said it. Without amusement.

So whom was I talking to? Not a whole person. For days she had lain in her hospital bed fluctuating between consciousness and unconsciousness, opening her eyes and closing them again. A tube had been pushed up through her nose and down into her stomach to feed her.

"I knew you didn't want any special efforts to be made for her," said Doctor Blake, just back from his vacation. "That is why this is such a distressing situation to be in." And then he made it clear that I would have to move her out of the hospital as soon as possible. Her crisis was over. Hospitals are not meant to handle slow, inevitable deaths. I hadn't prepared for that; I hadn't thought beyond the hospital, but in a daily encounter I held off Doctor Blake and the hospital administrative office until a bed was available back at the Bethesda Nursing Home.

Three weeks after Marko entered George Washington University Hospital, I called the ambulance to take her back to Bethesda. By nine in the morning she was rolled out into the noisy hospital corridor on a hard, narrow trolley. I couldn't make out what she was mumbling, but her wide eyes held me and I stood waiting with her, reassuring her as aides clattered metal basins, ran floor polishers and carried linens up and down the halls. At 11.20 the ambulance came and we made the return trip through Rock Creek Park.

"Remember me?" said Mrs Wines, the Admissions Director, coming into the lobby to greet her.

"Of course I do," replied Marko haughtily from her stretcher. She could still deflect a question to cover up her inability to remember a face or name. Then the ambulance men carried her into the Skilled Care Wing that I had so dreaded her ever entering. Her roommate, Mrs Stern, was blind and speechless, a former musician cut down by a stroke eight years earlier. Their room contained two beds, two night tables, two chairs and built-in chests of drawers for each patient. Yellow, delicately patterned wallpaper, soft lights, gold curtains, plants on the tables and windowsills and a fruit tree outside the window softened the spare furnishings.

But would Marko notice any of this? A doctor had explained that the injury to her right occipital lobe "blackened" or obscured the left half of her visual range. She could see only the right half of any objects or scenes she focused on. How strange it must seem to her who looked so hard and observed so closely to see only half of my face peering down at her. No wonder her expression was so intent. Usually after weeks or months some sort of compensation mechanism develops so that the victim slowly regains a full range of vision. With Marko we never knew if this happened because even though she retained her speech, her TIAs had caused diffuse cerebral lesions, so that she had what is termed "semantic aphasia". That is, she had progressively suffered a reduction in her capacity to speak in complex terms or to comprehend any complex ideas. This is a common phenomenon of senility. Her language generally was scaled down to simple expressions. Like Sir Walter Scott who sustained a series of strokes over a number of years, Marko retained her courtesy and social niceties. "How good of you to come," she'd say, or, "Thank you for your thoughtfulness".

But, because brain damage is highly selective, response patterns are not always consistent. Frequently stroke victims startle one with their intelligent awareness of what is going on or by their sudden ability to describe their feelings. Nurses, aides, and old friends crowded back into Marko's room welcoming her back. A frail white-haired woman from her poetry class leaned over her bed to ask plaintively, "Margaret, where *have* you been?"

With a deep sigh Marko replied, "I've been over the Alps." And then she closed her eyes, perhaps to re-enter that alpine landscape visible only to her and which I hoped was full of the grassy meadows dotted with blue and yellow wildflowers, sun-dappled snow-capped mountain peaks and sweet-smelling pines that she had known in her youth.

For several days after her move back to the nursing home she slept exhausted, in a near comatose state. She lay on a pliable water mattress. Aides awakened her and moved her limbs in passive exercises to keep her joints flexible. They propped her up in bed and her head lolled to the left. She pulled at the feeding tube in her nose. One day as I was filing her fingernails I remembered how she used to sew for me, her hands so quick and sure she could make me a dress in an afternoon. She always skipped the basting step and invariably forgot to pull out all the pins so that a date putting his arm around my waist might be scratched by a straight pin sticking out of a seam. More than once I accused her of deliberately loading me with fortifications. She would laugh and shrug and say, "Why not? You are my only daughter." Smiling at the memory I looked up at her silent, staring face and said, "You've always been a good mother." Immediately she replied, "It has always been my wish to be so." It was as if a stuffed likeness of Marko had spoken.

Stacy took the night train from Boston and Scott picked her up at Union Station at 8 am on a cold Thanksgiving morning. We took yellow chrysanthemums to Marko. Her eyes opened very wide and shone warmly with clear signals of recognition when she saw Stacy. Above her bed was still taped the sign, 'Nothing by Mouth,' and the feeding tube was still up her nose. A wince of pain flashed across Stacy's face when she saw them. "Dear Marko," she said, blowing in her ear and kissing her on the neck the way Marko used to do to her when she was small, "you are so handsome and you smell so sweet." Together we helped the nurse lift Marko out of bed and into a chair. The nurse put her bathrobe on backwards, strapped her in with a harness and placed her dark, puffy, paralysed left arm onto a pillow. She slumped to the left, unable to hold herself up, her neck limp as a rag doll's so that her head flopped to the side. She was as pathetic looking as any of the other paralytic, crippled and senile patients in the Skilled Care Wing — one of the ancient horrors I had hoped never to be near.

Tenderly Stacy brushed her hair and chatted about college. "I've had a piece of my sculpture chosen for an art show." "What kind?" Marko wanted to know.

On Christmas Day Bill, Scott, Stacy and I took her poinsettias. "You're looking much better," Bill said.

"I try to make myself think that I am," Marko whispered. We all heard her.

"She screws up her face like a baby when she yawns," Stacy observed, "and she sort of gurgles like babies do when they're snug and comfortable."

"She's reached a plateau. Don't expect any improvement," Doctor Blake advised. "We'll see," the nurses said. She was on no medication.

On 31 December I planted eight pots of blue and white hyacinths and wondered if Marko, the gardener, would be alive to see them bloom.

In mid-January her nose feeding tube was removed. She began to eat soft foods and stay awake longer. On 25 January Ellen and Watson sent red roses for her eighty-seventh birthday. Marko's eyes sparkled. "Not bad for an old gal, am I?" She smiled lopsidedly.

"By God, she *is* tough," Doctor Blake declared.

I wheeled her into the TV room where fifteen or twenty patients sat in a semicircle waiting to be fed from trays. Greedily some of the women reached out to touch me, crying, "Here I am, here, here. Hello. Here!" Mrs Stern, Marko's roommate, caught my hand and kissed it. Marko appeared not to notice any of them. I spooned custard into her mouth the way I had fed my babies, wiping what drooled out of the corners. Because of cranial nerve damage, food accumulated in the left side of her mouth and it bothered her.

Bill sat on the stool beside me next to Marko's wheelchair. "There are all women in here. No men," he observed. "Yes, there are," Marko mumbled. "They're out with the nurses."

"She's right," Bill said. "There are four men. All

of them sitting out there by the nurses' station. I wonder why?"

"Because men always get special treatment. They're the nurses' pets," Marko answered sharply. It was the first real feeling she had shown since her strokes. Bill and I looked at each other in amazement.

By mid-February she was eating solid foods, mumbling less and talking more, sometimes long, urgent monologues weaving back and forth across the loom of her life in a pattern too intricate for me always to follow. Frowning and fingering the crocheted afghan rug across her knees, she said, "They put these things around old ladies. Mama and Papa are in heaven. Clarence and Tom too. I haven't heard from Corinne in a long time. Can't wait to get my hands into some clay. Mother never got herself into a fix like I'm in now. Watch out. The Indians want your hair. Yes, Mama. I'll hide. Look out, look out! Sometimes I was a handful for Virgil. Don't fall off that log!" And she began to cry.

One day when Marko was sitting in her wheelchair with a foam rubber ring around her neck to keep her head from lolling over too far, she had a "petit mal", a small seizure. She was staring intently at me and had just said, "Where's Stacy?" when her eyes went vacant. She began to tremble, then shudder. Her eyes widened with a terrible look of helplessness and fear, then she lurched forward, her arms and legs jerked in a small spasm. Her face reddened.

"Please help me!" I called out to a nurse. But it was all over. With great gentleness the nurse and two aides lifted her back into bed. "Do you hurt?" "Do you have any pain?" they asked. "My back aches," Marko murmured.

"Would you like some ice cream?" She nodded yes. I watched her calmly accept spoonfuls of smooth ice cream. "She doesn't remember what happened," the nurse explained. "Patients never know they've had a seizure." The pain was mine. I fled to Jane's house. When she opened the front door I burst into tears. Without a question she took me straight up to her room, sat me in a rocking chair and brought me a tall, cold gin and tonic.

"Petit mals sometimes are preludes to severe strokes," Doctor Blake told me. And I knew that he hoped, as I did, that the next one would be final. She had two more seizures and the nurse called to say that with the last one she had sunk into a deep sleep. It was late February. After several storms the snow was piled high along the roadways. Bill and I finished dinner before we drove out through the snow-covered Rock Creek Park. Although Marko was still in the "deep sleep", some aura about her made me feel she was trying to respond. A nurse came in and lightly slapped her cheek saying, "Wake up, Mrs Smith." Marko scowled, jutting out her chin and pulling her mouth down at the corners. "You look just like Churchill, Margaret," Bill boomed at her. "Me?" She frowned and opened her eyes.

"Are you all right now?" I took her hand. She nodded faintly. "I didn't think I would ever be able to open my eyes."

"You tried very hard."

"Yes. I had to — my family."

"Does that include me?" Bill asked teasingly.

"You bet!" She said emphatically and moved her head in a trace of a nod. "You suit me as a son-in-law. It's such a pleasure when you ..." Her voice trailed off and she sank again into a fathomless sleep like a rock sinking down toward the dark ocean bed.

"If you ever want to see Marko again before she dies you better come pretty soon," I telephoned Watson. The dogwood was blooming all through the Park when I drove him and Ellen from the airport to the nursing home. Puffing on his unlit pipe, Watson declared, "This is one of the longest rides of my life."

I knew how much he dreaded seeing Marko so crippled and demented. Aloud, he wondered if she would recognise him. He and Ellen waited in the lobby while I went to see if Marko was ready. She had her hair freshly set. Somehow the aides had managed to get her into her best gold chiffon dress for the occasion. Her brown and yellow mohair throw rug was tucked up to cover her twisted leg and the harness holding her into the wheelchair. In the crook of her arm was her doll, Samantha, with a poke bonnet and a prairie dress that I had bought for her long ago at the suggestion of a nurse in the French Wing when Marko had her room there. Samantha kept Marko company. We had laughed over her and talked to her the way Marko and I had talked to my imaginary playmate when I was a little girl. She used to set a place at the table for my playmate even though Virgil scoffed. She and I understood the value of a neutral but always faithful friend of the imagination. When Marko came into the Skilled Care Wing a nurse had asked her where Samantha was and she replied with great dignity, "My daughter is keeping her at home." Now Samantha rested on and hid her paralysed arm.

But I had forgotten to tell Ellen and Watson about Samantha. It was painful enough to see Marko crippled in a wheelchair for the first time; a doll in her arm added too vivid a symbol of senility. A flicker of shock showed in their faces before they came forward with smiles. "Hi, Mom," Watson grinned, smoothing back his greying hair.

"Watsie! My darling baby boy!" She gave a cry of joy.

Muffling our guffaws, Ellen and I escaped behind her wheelchair. Watson shuffled from one foot to the other, laughing with us. "Gee, Mom," he fumbled. "You look great." Eagerly she reached out for him with her good right hand. His visit pulled her back and strengthened her tenacious hold on life.

In May I went on a tour to promote my book. Marko had "stabilised" again, as Doctor Blake said.

"That's not what's important," Jane declared. "What is important is that your and Bill's life goes on."

The hyacinths had bloomed and Stacy graduated from college in June and Marko was still alive.

# 11

# Let Her Pretend

One's life has value as long as one attributes value to the lives of others.

SIMONE DE BEAUVOIR: *The Coming of Age*

Slumped down in her wheelchair, Marko whispered, "I'm alive but it is very hard."

I wheeled her out onto the nursing home patio. Her eyes, pulled strongly to the right by the muscles of her non-paralysed side, nevertheless darted about. "Look at the trellis," she commanded. "The roses are beautiful." They were deep red, in full bloom, climbing up the trellis, crowding each other in glorious abundance. I sat on a bench and positioned her wheelchair close to the roses where she could catch their fragrance. "The sun feels good on my back," she murmured.

We had settled in for the long summer, sitting on the patio when I came to visit her. She was silent, staring intently. "What do you see, Marko?"

"A mountain."

"Is there snow on it?"

"Yes. It's beautiful."

Another long silence. "What do you see now?"

"A coyote."

"Is he big?"

"Oh, no. He could pass for a baby."

"Is he pretty?"

"Yes. Very. A beautiful animal. A lovely, deep beige."

"How lucky your mother is," the nurse said. "Prolonged hallucinations are common for people with dementia. But often they are frightening and paranoid. Mrs Smith is lucky to have such nice ones — in colour even."

But sometimes, looking anxiously over her shoulder, Marko saw Indians instead of beautiful mountains and handsome animals. "Where are the Indians?" I questioned her.

"All over the building. They're coming in everywhere. In the windows."

"What are you going to do?"

"Keep quiet."

"What do they want?"

"My hair." Her tone was matter-of-fact.

Other times she saw snakes. I knew they were the deadly "rattlers" she had learned to fear as a child come back to terrify her now. She had worn high-topped leather boots as protection against a surprise attack by a rattlesnake she might not see curled on a warm rock ready to strike if startled by her step. She had watched her mother cut the flesh to open wounds made by the rattler's fangs on the legs or arms of ranchers and helped her apply a suction cup to draw the venom out. Now she cried, "The snakes are there, on the ground. They're sliding towards me!"

"Don't worry. We'll go where there aren't any snakes. We'll be safe." I turned her wheelchair to push her to another room.

How vulnerable she was, how jumbled her world. She was the most pathetic looking patient of all those crowded into the social room for Friday afternoon's Happy Hour, her head sunk on her shoulder, her limp body held up in the chair by her harness. I looked around at the upright, ambulatory patients and hated them for being healthier than Marko. What did they know of pain and suffering?

Stroke patients cannot describe the physical sensations besetting them and there is a common misapprehension that strokes do not cause a painful condition. Testifying that that is not so, Guy Wint, a partially recovered stroke victim, wrote, "They [the doctors] could not grasp the physical stress shaking me; all its peculiar nature was hidden from them, and the compound of aches, pains and nervous sensations ... Always, the sense of concussion went on. Constant unremitting hammer blows ... The symptoms were kaleidoscopic. No sooner did the pain become easier in one limb than it appeared elsewhere in the body."

"Where do you hurt?" I asked Marko.

"Everywhere," she answered.

After his strokes, the poet Walt Whitman wrote that he felt as if his body were charged with an electric force. "I'm on fire," was what Marko moaned.

Winston Churchill's strokes caused his feet to itch insufferably. Marko complained, "The itching is driving me crazy."

Pain-killers helped but Marko could not always give a signal when she needed them. She wanted so little at this point: relief from her symptoms, to sit in the sun and to have some loved one near her. Yet she needed so much care it would be a misconception to think her life was simple. How often during that long hot summer I thought with longing of the slower-paced, simpler societies where aged relatives are kept at home sitting picturesquely on a bench in front of a white-washed house, the women with black scarves or white saris over their heads, smiling their toothless smiles, the men in caps sucking on unlit pipes. But who lifted them into bed and treated the sores worn on their haunches from so much sitting? Who washed their urine-stained clothes and changed their soaked bed linens? Who fixed their special soft foods and fed them? Washed their aged, aching limbs and rubbed them down with soothing lotions? Who watched them so they wouldn't eat straw or stray over the cliff? The servants in an Indian household. The many women in an extended village family.

The staff at the nursing home became my extended family. The West Indian aides told me about their grandmothers. Often they had been raised by these grandmothers. From them they learned to respect age. Their touch was gentle, their knowledge practical. They lifted Marko onto a stool on wheels and rolled her into the shower, rubbed her down with soft terry cloth towels, powdered her all over and soothed her limbs with lotions. "So refreshing," Marko smiled. Her face still brightened when I brought her new housecoats, one in apple green, another soft peach with a ruffled collar. She felt better when her hair was washed and curled.

"I'm making history," she said more than once, indicating she had some sense of beating the odds by being alive and that she derived pleasure from it. But one sultry day when her spirits were low she declared, "There's not much use in my staying around." To change the subject I mentioned that Stacy finally had found a job teaching art but felt a bit apprehensive of the prospect and Marko startled me by responding with a rare laugh. "I know. I was scared to death when I went to Lewiston Normal School. It was all I could do to keep from crying all week."

Somehow my remark had switched on her memory of how lonely and frightened she had been when as a young girl she had packed her saddle bags and ridden off from her parents' ranch to a new life of her own making. Some connection in her brain made her able to relate that first week at Normal School over sixty years ago to the apprehension felt by her granddaughter today.

She laughed again. "I guess I'll have to talk to Stacy."

But these flashes of contact were exceptional. Most of the time Marko mumbled incoherently or mouthed silently, occasionally enunciating a clear word or phrase unattached to any discernible meaning. Once in a while whole sentences and the fragments of conversations suddenly popped out which I seldom could find a context for. What was left of Marko's mind seemed to be connected with her distant past that I knew so little about. Listening to her reminded me when, years ago when Bangladesh was East Pakistan, I had sat before a shortwave radio straining hungrily to hear newscasts relayed from home. But I seldom caught more than a few suggestive words and tantalising phrases through the static and interference. Now I was seized with a yearning to know more about my mother who uttered her isolated signals sitting here before me in her old woman's body — a body so familiar to me but that she had lived in only a short part of her life. I knew its every intimate detail, the sturdy feet whose toenails I cut, the slim ankles I rubbed with lotion, the long appendectomy scar on her sagging belly, the smooth white back and wrinkled neck, patrician nose and high forehead.

But the young Margaret Watson whom I had never met lived in a slim-waisted, high-bosomed body I knew only from pictures. She stood smiling in a knitted cap with ice-skates hanging over her shoulder or sat in front of her basketball team in the full-bloomered uniform of the captain, a bow in her hair, a basketball in her lap, or looked serious astride a sleek horse, holding the reins in her gloved hands, her riding jacket nipped tightly at her waist. She was a stranger about whom I had heard stories. Now it was the stranger I wanted to know.

A few times she mistook Pat Lax, who still faithfully visited her, for me. "I'm so tired," she confided to Pat.

One day when she felt stronger she declared vehemently, "If I could, I would cut out this part of my life and just hang it on the wall."

I wrote down every comprehensible utterance that burst through her unintelligible ramblings as if I were collecting the last blossoms from a dying tree, faded and fragile blooms, but unmistakable signs of life to show my friends and family. "Don't get obsessed," warned Jane Weld. "You have other obligations — to yourself, to Bill, the boys and Stacy."

In the fall Marko caught a cold and ran a fever of 102°F. Lying in bed she looked so pale and drawn. "Would you like something to drink?" I asked. "Maybe some ginger ale?"

A faint light came into her eyes. "How about some alcohol?" she whispered.

In December I wheeled her into the lobby to see the Christmas tree. From a distance of about twenty-five feet she said with scorn,"It's artificial." Up closer she noted,"It needs something around the bottom."

On 23 December Marko had another "episode". She turned quite green around the nose and mouth and stopped breathing for about fifteen seconds. The nurse gave her a whiff of oxygen and she rallied. Like Queen Elizabeth I with all of her court around her watching and waiting, she wouldn't die.

Stacy sat with me beside Marko's bed on Christmas Eve. For a long time Marko didn't recognise her. About three or four times she seemed to focus intently on the far distance with a peaceful expression we had never seen before. Her face was shiny and waxen. Once Stacy got up to get a Kleenex. When she turned her back Marko saw her in the mirror across the room and murmured, "There's Stacy." Then she appeared to stop breathing. A great stillness seemed to settle over her. Except for the slow, throbbing pulse in her neck we would have thought she had died. "Watch her throat," I whispered to Stacy. She nodded. Each of us held one of her hands, hardly daring to breathe, fearful of death but hoping it would come when we were there and she knew we were holding her hands.

Hours passed. Her cheeks puffed smoother still with the fluids her heart was not beating strongly enough to carry away. Her face glossed with sweat. Her eyes closed and finally we left.

The next day was the second Christmas since Marko's massive stroke. She lifted her head when we all came with presents of cologne and slippers and the chocolates she loved. The waxy look and smooth puffiness in her face were gone, leaving her cheeks sunken and dark circles around her eyes. She had been to the brink and back once again.

"When I was little I had no one to bring me things," she said in a whisper. Could she know it was Christmas? She reached out to pull down my sleeve and straighten my scarf, the urge to improve me still alive in her.

And so it went on through January, past her eighty-eighth birthday, my life bound to the ups and downs of hers. I did her washing to save on laundry bills, shopped for hard-to-find clothes that would be comfortable, kept her accounts and worried about money. Each time I went to see her I hoped she would say something witty or revealing for me to write down in my notebook and repeat to my family and friends. "You're getting too tired," Jane cautioned me. "It's foolish."

I might have been trying to make up for all those years I had lived overseas so far away from her, for the sins of omission I felt towards her, or perhaps I was suffering from a belated guilt for not fully appreciating her strengths. Now she had slowed down my life so that sitting long hours beside her I began to reflect on how different her life was from mine — a truism I had of course always known intellectually, but never had fleshed out emotionally. Slowly there came to me a realisation of the ingenuity, effort and self-discipline required by her to build such a broad, rich life for Watson and me, starting as she had from a spare, hard frontier existence. She kindled these thoughts the day she surprised me by saying with a wonderful little laugh and twinkle in her voice, "Whoever would have thought when I was living up on the Joseph Plain that I would be stopping in London? I liked London."

Later she grabbed my hand. "I want to tell you, read!" she said urgently.

"Read what?"

She looked at me vacantly. Then something connected and she murmured, "Get inspiration in great books."

But I think that basically what kept pulling me back to sit patting her hand and listening for clues to the woman I now wished I knew better was a simple love and a strong curiosity. I was no more dedicated than members of other families. I came to visit Marko less often than the son of her roommate, Mr Stein, who stopped in to see his mother every day and had done so for eight years, or than other people who, far from deserting their wives or husbands, mothers or fathers in the nursing home, remained faithfully attentive. For me there was a compelling fascination that at such an advanced stage of dementia and physical deterioration, such sparks of originality could still fly from Marko. I smiled at her and she smiled back. "We make faces at each other," she said. "It's hard to know what to do," she so aptly observed as bit by bit she continued to disintegrate, to disconnect.

Sometimes she was fidgety and cross. I brought her a bunch of pansies, remembering how she used to grow them and liked to point out to me the marvellous variety of markings on their faces.

"Here are some pansies, Marko. Do you like them?"

"No."

"Why not?"

"They grow too close to the ground."

All the time she was rolling her eyes, looking hard. "Some people," she muttered, her jaw tightening, a look of disapproval settling on her face.

"Some people what?"

"Open their mouths."

Across the lounge from her was a skeleton of an old man asleep with his mouth open. She was offended. I wheeled her across the hall. "OK?" I asked. "That's fine," she replied, her face relaxing.

One Sunday when she was particularly clear-minded, she told Bill that she liked him better without his glasses, so he took them off and put them in his lap. With her good right hand she reached over, picked them up, shook the frames open, put them on and screwed up her eyes, blinking rapidly.

"Why did you do that, Margaret?" Bill asked.

"Oh, I don't know. Just to be funny, I guess." And she laughed. "You know, Bill," she added, "you are becoming a great comfort to the family."

"I note your tense," Bill said, "becoming," and he hugged her. She beamed at him.

"You raised a fine daughter," he told her.

Marko looked away and was silent. We thought we had lost contact with her. Then she replied very seriously, "I worked hard on her."

Comments like that kept me bound to her through all the bad days when she made no sense whatsoever. Once when she seemed restless, as if she wanted something, I enquired, "Would you like a chocolate? Are you hungry?"

"All the time." She raised her eyebrows and we laughed at our private, long-standing joke that nothing ever interfered with our appetites. Even with raging fevers or broken bones we could always enjoy a good meal.

"I wish Virgil would come by," she sighed as I adjusted her neck brace.

Bill and Scott spelled me on my Wednesday and weekend visits when they could. I was feeling more and more drained. Often Marko was in bed now, too tired to be up very long in her wheelchair. "When spring comes we'll all feel better," she had said when I complained about the snow. Now, in May, she lay on her side, so small and still under the sheet, not moving when I greeted her. I bent down and she puckered her mouth through the safety bars on the side of her bed for me to kiss her. Her face was contorted as if she were going to cry. She was talking to herself in an anguished tone, gibberish sounding until finally I heard her say, "I haven't accomplished enough."

"But Marko, you have," I assured her. "You've done so much. You've worked so hard and been so busy all your life."

"No," she wept. "Mother says, 'Get busy. You've been idle long enough. Get to work. You've wasted enough time.'" And she sobbed inconsolably. I tried to distract her, to make her laugh, but she was the little girl whose mother was angry with her for reading the newspapers she was supposed to be lining the kitchen cupboards with and for escaping to the outhouse to dream over the possibilities of another life tantalisingly suggested by the illustrations in the Sears Roebuck catalogue.

What made her remember those scoldings? Without discernible stimulus her mind ground on, throwing up snatches of memories loaded with all of the emotional freight the original experience evoked. Another time she remembered a small kindness done her forty years before. "I told Mrs Galloway I needed pots for my plants and she said, 'You wait, you'll get them.' And she got them for me." Her face glowed.

I hadn't heard Mrs Galloway's name since I was a very small child, when Marko would have been a young wife living in the big colonial house near the University of Washington in Seattle. She and Virgil moved from Boise, Idaho, when Watson was six and into their own house shortly before I was born. "Which corner of which room do you want me to put your furniture?" the mover had asked them.

In a sudden shift of mood she clung to my hand and rasped, "I'm so glad you're here with me. I'm not alone, am I?" How could I leave her?

"You've got to take a vacation," Jane said. Bill was planning a canoe trip for us down the Yukon River with our old friends, Jane and Carl Coon. It seemed an impossibility to me. "I love you," I told her and wiped away the little line of spittle drooling out of the paralysed side of her mouth.

"We like each other," she replied. Then after a moment she added, "And we are justified in doing so."

But sometimes when I came to see Marko there was no response in her eyes. Her blank stare was unnerving. I was not sure she really knew me. Whatever loving responses I eventually elicited from her might be for anyone. Greedily I prompted her to give me a sign of recognition, to say my name, and always she did.

Then on the night of Friday, 13 June, 1980, Mount St Helens, near Seattle, activated by the intense lunar pull, erupted again. And Marko had another stroke.

"She's just like the mountain, keeping us all wondering when the next eruption will be," said Blair, calling from Seattle.

Within thirty-six hours Marko was sitting up in her wheelchair wearing her pale peach housecoat with the ruffle at the neck. But there was a significant change in her expression — a terrible, total blankness that had not been there before. For the first time a stroke had occurred in the left hemisphere of her brain so that now her right side was flaccid, or nearly so, as already she was regaining some motor control in her right arm.

"It's me. Luree." I held her face in my hands and called to her. "Marko, it's me. Your daughter."

"She didn't come home for lunch," was all she would say.

Desperately I cajoled and beseeched her to recognise me. A nurse tried to make her respond and Bunny, the aide she liked best, kept repeating, "Come on now, Mrs Smith, who is this? You know her." Once she replied, "Ethel Frank," a name I didn't recognise. Finally, exasperated by Bunny's prodding, she gave an imperious little wave with her good right hand and said with impatient finality, "Oh, let her pretend to be whoever she wants to be." I backed away, staring at the bland expression on her face, at her big brown, vacant eyes. Then I turned and bolted from her room, ran down the hall and hid behind the nurses' station sobbing like a child.

"Now you must go," Jane declared. "If she dies while you're gone I'll be here to help Scott. He can call me immediately and I'll go with him."

"It's healthier to see the body," Mrs Wines, the Admissions Director, advised me. "Otherwise the death does not seem real. But don't worry. Mrs Smith will be here when you get back. At the rate she is going she may outlive us all."

## 12

# MARGARET, HOW I WISH I KNEW YOU

Tell me the tales that to me were so dear,
Long, long ago, long, long ago.

THOMAS HAYNES BAYLY: *Long, Long Ago*

Several more days passed and still Marko gave no sign of recognising me. The last evening before I left for the Yukon she lay in her bed in her ruffled peach housecoat, her white hair brushed back in a deep wave off her forehead. With her great brown eyes benignly blank she stared at me, then her eyelids began to droop drowsily.

"Goodbye, Marko," I said, bending down to kiss her.

"Goodbye, darling," she answered automatically with a small sleepy smile. I didn't press her to say more. All of my hopes for recognition from her were dead. I stood at the doorway of her spare room watching her regular breathing, her peaceful sleep.

Inexplicably I still felt reluctant to leave.

But once I was airborne over the Great Plains and higher still crossing the Rocky Mountain range, I began to feel a weight and tension of responsibility give way to a bone tiredness. Jane had been right. I had become obsessed with Marko. It is a common phenomenon among caretakers of elderly parents or spouses, particularly if the afflicted person is suffering from dementia, to be convinced they never can leave their sides. Somehow one cannot quite believe that the mind of a loved one is coming apart. Irrational hope that the process will reverse or cease and stabilise at a functional level keeps the caretaker riveted to that person, watching, hoping against all that they know, against all the advice and counsel of doctors and friends, for a change for the better that never comes.

Sometimes as caretakers we see what isn't there, grasp at signs of rationality that may be nothing more than empty reflexes. How often in the last two years Marko really knew me I'll never be certain. Whether my brushing her hair, rubbing her legs or wheeling her on to the patio made her any happier than when a nurse's aide did the same thing I'll never know.

Shortly before I went West with Bill and the Coons, Jane Weld told me a story full of warnings. A friend of hers, in her late middle years, suddenly found herself faced with the care of her invalid mother. Her mother had been quite independent, living some distance from her, when a stroke left her bedridden and mentally incompetent. Jane's friend was so devastated by this catastrophic development that she brought her mother to live with her until her husband, at his retirement, finally convinced her that the mother's care was too much of a burden at home and so she placed her in a nursing facility nearby. Twice a day she went to the nursing home to feed her mother. This self-imposed duty prevented her from travelling or taking part in other activities with her husband and friends. Two years after her husband retired her mother died. Six months later her husband was dead. She was a widow whose friends had long since ceased to call her.

Jane's point was well taken, I thought, as we launched our canoes in the headwaters of the Yukon River. Life must go on. I had become dull and driven, focusing so intently on Marko's slow decline. Acceptance of the inevitable never has been easy for me. Perhaps this stubborn, irrational belief that you can overcome almost any obstacle is an attitude typical of the frontier West. Contemplating the rugged wilderness around me I began to muse on what incorrigible optimists my forebears must have been to have come West when they did. They were spirited people given more to action than introspection, and already, as I dipped my paddle in the cold, clear water, stroking hard, I felt better. Even though I knew only the barest bones about them, their very coming across the Rockies bequeathed to me a sense of belonging in the woods and mountains so restoring to the spirit.

Marko's grandfather, Perry Watson, and his bride, Mary Jane Needham, were part of the great western migration that began in the 1840s. In 1849 they left Kentucky and crossed the Great Plains on the Oregon Trail in a covered wagon to homestead near Salem, Oregon. Perry's son Tom married my Swiss grandmother, Louisa Tuescher and they had six children. The first three, Clarence, Margaret and Tom, Jr, were born in Oregon. "Papa was a deputy sheriff and drove a stagecoach drawn by six beautiful matched dapple-grey horses," Marko had often told me. Invariably she added that when her father rode into town shouting and cracking his whip over the horses' backs she and her brothers would run out to meet him nearly bursting with pride and excitement.

But like so many pioneers, Tom Watson was restless and found town life too confining. So he moved his family across the Snake River to Idaho, up through the primeval forests to the high Joseph Plain, in the Salmon River Mountains where he homesteaded, raised horses and led pack trains to the silver mines at Buffalo Hump and other mining strikes. On that isolated ranch Marko learned to bake bread, make soap and candles, break horses, and be alert for signs of storms or mountain lions or unfriendly Indians.

Sitting around our campfires in the Yukon wilderness, I thought of Marko riding her horse through the mountains of Idaho. Here it was easy to imagine her as a girl and a young woman, to conjure pictures of her to ameliorate the bitter, sharp, immediate memories of her slouched and vacant-eyed in her wheelchair. Although she was not yet dead, I had been mourning her for nearly ten years since the day she collapsed and Watson took her to the hospital. Now I was beginning the final healing process, sorting out the memories I wanted to preserve, reaching back to the heritage I wanted to rescue from the morass of bad times we had just been through.

I remember asking her when I was small, "Weren't you ever scared when you were alone in the mountains?" "Not if I had a good horse," she would reply in a reckless tone, with a light in her eyes. "Give a good horse his head and he'll never lead you into trouble — unless, of course, he sees a rattler or smells smoke." And then she would tell me the story of the time she and Clarence were caught on the down-wind side of a fire raging through a forest of dry yellow pines; how they soaked their clothes in a stream to protect themselves from the heat, blindfolded her skittish horse, and with Clarence clutching her reins they raced to safety.

Why couldn't I remember more? Marko told me stories all through my childhood and now when they would mean so much, most of them had slipped away from me. When I was an adolescent I was too narcissistic to take note of her life and during the long period it took me to grow up I fell, like most daughters (and sons), into the fruitless pattern of maligning and blaming her (and my father to a lesser extent) for most of my own problems. Then one day I forgave her for not being perfect. I can't remember just when I bestowed my forgiveness on her, but somewhere in my twenties or thirties it began to sink into my consciousness that I might be, in my own way almost, though of course not quite, as fallible as she.

"The older we get the more we appreciate our mothers," a woman in one of my writing classes had remarked, and the simple wisdom of this statement attracted me the more I thought about it. But how can we appreciate them, how can we imagine the worlds our mothers lived in, worlds that changed so quickly and so radically that it is next to impossible to understand what they had to cope with as they grew up?

After our canoe trip I went back to that still remote part of Idaho to see if I could discover some sense of what it had been like in the early part of the century when Marko lived there. But the road up to the ranch on the Joseph Plain is impassable now. No one lives in that inaccessible area where Marko's sister Corinne was born, the first white baby to be born between the Snake and Salmon Rivers. She came prematurely, just as the family, with their loaded wagons, started moving down from the high summer pasture. While Tom Jr and Clarence drove the horses back into the corral, Marko helped open the cabin they had closed up for the winter. Her anxious father disappeared into the bedroom with her mother and shouted to Marko to light the stove for heat and water, and to find a box and fill it with fluffed-up cotton for the tiny baby they had not expected to arrive until they were settled at home in their permanent ranch house at a lower elevation.

Was that the memory Marko's mind clung to, making her cry out from her wheelchair, "Is Mama all right? Is Mama all right?"

Two more girls came later, so there were four: Margaret, Corinne, Luree and Louise, the four Watson beauties with their clear, glowing complexions and their tiny corseted waists. They rode for miles to dances in the one-room school buildings or grange halls, dancing the night through, then piling into their father's wagon to drive home as the sun rose over the Bitterroot Mountains to the east.

They all were great mimics and story-tellers and laughed with wonderful abandon. I loved to listen to them sitting around a kitchen table drinking coffee and telling stories. "Tell me about Charlie," I would beg. Their best stories were about their beaus, and Charlie was one who pursued them all, a hayseed they said, who wore yellow boots and red suspenders. He loved to dance. Once Charlie had grasped one of them by the waist with his huge rough hand and with the other hand hoisted hers, straight-armed like a signal for battle: there was no escape as he charged down the hall. Marko and one of her sisters would get up to demonstrate. When they reached the end of the room Marko would shout through her nose in an imitation of Charlie's nasal voice, "Reverse, sweetheart, reverse!" and she and her partner would sweep, stiff-legged, back again.

Often when I wheeled Marko around at the end of the nursing home hall to push her back to her room, I would bend down to say in a nasal voice, "Reverse, sweetheart, reverse," and sometimes she would smile.

In Lewiston, Idaho, I looked for but couldn't find the Normal School where in 1913 Marko received her certificate to teach — her passport to independence and escape from the strenuous life on the ranch where time to read or draw had to be stolen. Summers when she could be spared she helped with the cooking and dishwashing on other ranches to earn money to go to school. Small wonder that she was so mystified later on when one of Watson's daughters chose for a while to live in the woods, cook on a wood stove and raise and can fruits and vegetables. It had been from just such a tyranny of mind-dulling toil that Marko had fled.

She became one of those pioneering young women of the West who went off to live in boarding houses in little frontier towns and teach eight grades in one-room schoolhouses. In a picture I have, taken in front of her first school in White Bird, Idaho, she is standing beside her twenty-eight pupils, a half-dozen of them taller than she is. Her white, stiffly starched, long-sleeved, high-collared blouse is tucked into her dark, ankle-length skirt, her hair brushed back from her high forehead, her face serious with the responsibilities of her position. Teachers in those days held an important, prestigious place in the community. They had standards to uphold. Once Marko rode pillion on a dashing suitor's motor cycle the length of Main Street and was lectured by the School Board and the minister for conduct unbecoming to a teacher.

Marko met Virgil at a summer teacher's institute in Moscow, Idaho. A graduate of the University of Missouri Law School, he had left a law practice to come West to pursue his original ambition to teach. When, on holidays, he rode over from Ferdinand where he first taught, to court Marko, her brothers teased her about this "Easterner" who didn't know how to sit a horse. Although all of the Watson girls were short like their mother, Clarence and Tom Jr, like their father, were over six feet tall. Hawk-nosed, barrel-chested and bronzed as Indians, they rode bucking broncos and wrestled steers by their horns to the ground in local fairs and rodeos. Marko adored them but she shared the same dreams as Virgil.

I stood at the top of White Bird Hill and gazed over the magnificent panorama of wild and uninhabited hills where the Nez Perce Indians and the US Cavalry had fought their bloody battles, hills peaceful now, dotted only with stands of dark green pines. Directly below the lookout point, a full mile down, I could see the little town of White Bird, a double line of yellow or white frame buildings, some nearly hidden from view by clumps of silvery green cottonwoods, strung along the curve of the Salmon River. It was the only habitation in sight. At the top of the hill the wind blew fresh and clear, its lonely murmur the only sound under the huge blue dome of sky. The marker by the side of the road read: "Salmon River: A vast mountain wilderness, cut by the mile-deep Salmon River Canyon, stretches across Idaho South and East of here. Travel through the Salmon River mountains always was hard in the early days. An 1872 railway survey showed the Salmon River canyon to be too expensive a route to build. Until a highway was finished down White Bird Hill in 1921, only some pack trails and a difficult wagon road crossed the rugged mountain barrier that separates north and south Idaho."

In 1913 Marko crossed this mountain barrier, riding from the north down White Bird Hill to her first teaching post. She stayed two years. Her happy memories of that time, of ice-skating on the Salmon River, building great bonfires to warm by, and sitting down to eat meals at Mrs Rigg's boarding house that she didn't have to cook or wash up after, stayed with Marko over all the years so that at the nursing home a skilled writing teacher was able to coax out of her poems about them.

In 1915 she moved to another school at Stites on the South Fork of the Clearwater River. She kept on drawing and carving in wood and went to summer school sessions at the University of Idaho. She made her own clothes, tutored pupils on the side and dreamed of art school in Berkeley at the University of California. When she had enough money to go, Virgil jumped on the same train and rode all the way to California with her. There is a picture in her album of the two of them in Golden Gate Park in 1916. Marko is wearing a smartly tailored suit, the skirt reaching to the top of her shoes, her large straw hat tilted jauntily to one side, and she is smiling broadly. Virgil is looking at her, his face shadowed by his felt fedora. That year she married the persistent lawyer from the 'East', later bore Watson, then me, and no longer being mistress of her fate, reshaped her dreams.

The night before we flew home from our canoe trip I made one last call to Scott for a report on Marko. She had been sleeping a lot, he told me. Then almost imperceptibly she slipped into a coma, he said, and just five hours before I called, she had died. All day the nurses and aides had stopped in to hold her hand and give her comfort and assurance.

"Marko's timing was perfect," Jane had told Scott when she met him at the nursing home. "She died just before Luree got home — a last present to her." Together Jane and Scott went into Marko's room. "It wasn't hard to see her," Scott said. "She was in her own bed and looked very peaceful with her eyes closed. Her skin was very smooth." He kissed her on the forehead and then Jane kissed her for all of us.

Marko was eighty-eight years and seven months old when she died. But for me those last years of her distress were already dimming in the great healing sense of space and tranquillity that I found in the mountains of the West. Instead of remembering her poor limp body and lolling head, I focused in my mind's eye the fresh, open face of Margaret Watson of Joseph, Idaho, wearing her riding pants and chaps, a perky bow tie at the collar of her high-necked blouse, sitting easily in her saddle. Because I had been there I can imagine the young teacher who sent her trunk ahead by wagon and rode her horse confidently, giving it its head, down the switchback trail on White Bird Hill, out into a world full of learning and adventure. Before it began to go, nearly sixty years later, my mother's mind was bright and eager and that is what I must remember.

# 13

# AFTERWARDS THE ASHES

I am a part of all that I have met.

ALFRED, LORD TENNYSON: *Ulysses*

"Exactly what should I expect when I come to pick up my mother's ashes?" I asked the woman who answered the phone at the funeral home.

"A brown sealed plastic box heavier than you might imagine," she said. "A body burns down to about five pounds of ashes. And if you're going to scatter them I should tell you that not all of the bones burn completely. There will be some pieces."

Forearmed with that information I picked up the heavy plastic box on a hot August day and put it beside me on the front seat of the car. I had a strong sense of Marko's presence, a surprisingly good feeling. She was with me again. My obligation to her was not quite over — her ashes had to be scattered as she had instructed me. At home I tucked the box in the big rosewood chest she and I had found at Chor Bazaar in Bombay until the time I could take it to Seattle.

"Don't leave her there too long. Don't postpone it," a friend told me a few weeks later as we were riding the crowded Metro. "It's amazing how you can put such things off and forget." She warmed to her subject. "I was cleaning out the attic the other day and came across Uncle Bert and he's been dead twenty years at least." Eyes swivelled our way. I assured her that I wouldn't forget and leave Marko's ashes in the rosewood chest.

First, to inform scattered friends and family of her death I sent out a four by six inch folded paper with her dates, 25 January 1892, to 22 August 1980, on the front and two snapshots of her taken in the Blue Ridge Mountains shortly before her strokes, one in her picture hat in front of a dogwood tree, her expression intent, and the other with her head thrown back, laughing with that infectious abandon. Inside I wrote, "In her mid-eighties Margaret said, 'I've had an interesting life. I've done a lot. I've been to a lot of places and I've seen a lot of things. It's been a good life and you must not be sad when I die. I'm ready and I'm not scared. Remember that!'"

"We do," I wrote. "Watson, Luree and their families have a great legacy of memories," and then I sketched a quick summary of her life.

Rather than memorial services, Watson and I decided to have memorial dinners, his on the West Coast and mine on the East, spanning the continent she so loved to travel across. Ellen and I each set our tables with care, using the linen and dishes Marko left us. With our respective families and friends we drank toasts to her, told stories and reminisced. "What I remember," said Stacy, "is that Marko always had faith in me. It was great to have a grandmother like that. I always knew that no questions asked, Marko would go to the wall for me." Had Marko been able to hear Stacy's testimony, she would have narrowed her eyes fiercely, her clan instincts aroused, wagged her finger and said, "You bet I would!"

Then Scott read one of the poems Marko loved, Tennyson's "Ulysses", and we sang, as rousingly as we could, some of her favourite songs that she used to pound out on the piano: "When It's Springtime in the Rockies", "Red River Valley", and "Drink to Me Only With Thine Eyes". She came back to us in all her rich diversity and Jane, with her gift for the comforting phrase, said, "You did everything you could to support her and she did everything she could to support you." To some extent that was true. But like all mothers and daughters we often fell short of the expectations we had for each other. Very reluctantly I became Marko's caretaker — I had wanted her to remain strong and independent to the end. Once I finally accepted the fact that she couldn't help what was happening to her, I belatedly took up my obligation to see her through. In a way she had done the same for me, seeing me through a childhood different from what she no doubt dreamed of for her only girl. In many ways I was not the daughter she had hoped I would be: I was not interested in the things she was interested in and was devoid of an artistic talent she could nurture.

A letter of condolence from Christy, my old school friend, unintentionally carried that sharp reminder. "I remember," Christy wrote, "sitting on the floor of your mother's bedroom, leaning against the *chaise longue*, Margaret standing at the ironing board, pressing hems with a damp cloth and listening to her lecture on the mysteries of facings and inner facings, of tailor's padding and the right 'marriage of fabric' and watching the magic she created work itself before my eyes." I was impervious to that magic and probably at the time was out playing baseball. Daughters (and sons) seldom do what their mothers hope most for them. Marko gave up trying to teach me to draw or paint or sew or garden. Parents and children move through the same world seeing it with such different perspectives, responding with different talents and abilities, it is small wonder that they often feel they have failed each other. But the bond of familial love is tenacious, however frayed and knotted. In the end children must put their parents to rest, attend to the details of their deaths.

Nearly a year after Marko died, I slipped the box

of her ashes into my flight bag and took the plane to Seattle. Blair met me at the airport enthusiastic with the suggestion that I take his kayak out into Puget Sound to scatter her ashes that way. "I think Marko would like that." He beamed. "It would be different and she liked to do adventurous things. Think of it: she had tried just about every other mode of travel — horseback, wagon, buggy, cars, trucks, motor cycle, ferry boats, Watson's sailboat, ocean liners, trains, planes, camel, elephant, but I never had a chance to get her out in my kayak."

Imagining myself trying to manoeuvre the double-ended paddle to keep the kayak from going broadside and taking water in the frigid waves of Puget Sound, and at the same time trying to handle the five-pound box of ashes, I demurred.

But how to scatter her ashes was a problem. Watson and I considered tossing them from the end of one of the ferries she loved to ride, but dismissed that as too public. People might stare. We considered spreading them on the waves from the end of one of the piers along the Seattle waterfront where she used to set up her easel to paint the fishing boats or the snow-capped Olympic mountains across Puget Sound. But that too was a public place. Then it occurred to us what a beachcomber Marko had been. Walking barefooted on the sand at the tide-line, her pants rolled to her knees or her skirt tucked up in her belt, she bent down to pick up agates and unusual stones for her rock garden and paths and shells for her kitchen windowsills. Inspired by that remembrance we chose to take Marko's ashes to the quiet little beach at Carkeek Park tucked below the bluff her house was on, across from Agate Pass, that she could see from her living room windows.

We settled on a day in July when the tide was high: eleven feet six inches at 5.42 pm. The temperature was in the upper 60s, the air clear and fresh smelling after a light drizzle. The slanting rays of the setting sun lit the snowy peaks of the Olympics and traced shimmering streaks of light across the slate-green water of Puget Sound. Watson carried the box of Marko's ashes. Since it was sealed, he had tried to open it first at home with his tools, but being unable to pry the lid open, he resorted to boring two holes in the end and covering them with wide scotch tape. As we walked down through the tall grass we wondered how we would feel when we poured the ashes out. Dallying for time we picked the wild blackberries growing along the path, savouring their sweet taste, and pinched the salmon berries only to find them not yet ripe. Down on the beach we sat a while on a smooth, silvery log half buried in the sand and smelled the salty, pungent sea air that Marko had grown to love more than the scent of mountain pines. "She had some bad times, but she had more good times," Watson said.

We walked along the logs washed up on the beach and over the rocks looking for a suitable spot to empty the box. Where the beach swept around into a small cove we spotted a single, large grey-black granite rock. Small waves were breaking at its base and running back down the sand, strewing small rocks, pebbles and white lines of foam across the sand. "Perfect!" I exclaimed. "Marko would say that the rock looks like a huge turtle with its head up headed out to sea."

"Right," Watson said. "Cup your hands and I'll pour out some of her ashes." We looked at each other a moment and both of us took a deep breath. Watson gave me a quizzical grin. "Here goes." He pulled back the scotch tape and poured the fine, white ashes mixed with tiny pieces of chalk white bone into my hands. The bits of bone were like shards of bleached shells worn smooth by the waves and the ashes were so soft and light I could scarcely feel them. But there Marko was — all that was tangibly left of her there in my hands. Holding her delicate clean white ashes out in the fresh open air suddenly seemed so right. I felt a great wave of peacefulness, almost joy, sweep through me. I smiled at Watson. "Go ahead," he said. I stepped across the water line onto the back of the turtle rock, waited for a big wave and threw my handful of Marko's ash onto its crest. The wave broke in a salty white froth and rolled back, carrying her ashes out to mingle with the waters of Puget Sound. What she had wanted.

I leaped back to the shore and flung my arms around Watson, hugging him hard. "It's just right, absolutely right," I cried with relief.

"Okay, now you pour." He cupped his hands. And so, alternately, we tossed handfuls of Marko's ashes out to the sea until the last light traces of ash were lifted by the wind and none were left. Then as if some deep, primitive instinct rose simultaneously in both of us, we bent down to collect small shells and rocks from the spot where we had made our final parting with our mother. Such a simple spontaneous action made us smile and we hugged each other again. Somehow Marko had sensed that for us, her son and her daughter, to handle the last earthly traces of her ourselves completed a cycle in harmony with nature. This final act in Marko's long slow death released us. We had looked at death long and hard and found this ending good.

# Alzheimer's Association Addresses

Alzheimer's Association (Australia)
P.O. Box 51
North Ryde, NSW 2113
Tel: (02) 878 4466

NEW SOUTH WALES
Alzheimer's Association (NSW)
P.O. Box 42
North Ryde 2113
Tel: (02) 805 0100
HELP LINE 008 810 604

NORTHERN TERRITORY
Alzheimer's Association (NT)
c/- P.O. Box 38919
Winnellie 0821
Tel: (089) 22 742

QUEENSLAND
Alzheimer's Association (Qld)
P.O. Box 446
Lutwyche 4030
Tel: (07) 857 4043

SOUTH AUSTRALIA
Alzheimer's Association (SA)
P.O. Box 202
Eastwood 5063
Tel: (08) 373 2670

TASMANIA
Alzheimer's Association (TAS)
P.O. Box 1606
Hobart 7001
Tel: (002) 34 8884

VICTORIA
Alzheimer Society of Victoria
98 Riverside Road
Hawthorn 3122
Tel: (03) 818 3022

WESTERN AUSTRALIA
Alzheimer's Association (WA)
P.O. Box 1099
Subiaco 6008
Tel: (09) 388 2128